Confronting Life-Threatening Illness: Mind-Body Approaches

The paper used in this publication meets the minimum requirements
of American National Standard for Information Sciences—
Permanence of Paper for Printed Library Materials,
ANSI Z39.48-1984.

Confronting Life-Threatening Illness:
Mind-Body Approaches

Edited by Suzanne R. Engelman

Roger W. Bartrop
Thomas Baumann
Hans-Peter Bilek
Annegret Boll
Norman Cousins
Atle Dyregrov
Suzanne R. Engelman
Dirk Fehlenberg
Steven Fleck
Lina Forcier
Dan Hertz
Wolfgang Jacob
Michael Jones
Margit von Kerekjarto
Rudolf Klussman
Karl Köhle
Thomas Küchler
Ebbe Linnemann
Jeffrey T. Mitchell
Ronald Penny
Hubert Speidel
Reidar Thyholdt
Thure von Uexküll

❖

IRVINGTON PUBLISHERS, INC.
NEW YORK

Copyright © 1993 by Irvington Publishers, Inc.

All rights reserved. No part of this book may be reproduced in any manner whatever, including information storage, or retrieval, in whole or in part (except for brief quotations in critical articles or reviews), without written permission from the publisher.
Please address permission requests to
Irvington Publishers, Inc.,
740 Broadway, New York, New York 10003

Irvington Publishers, Inc.,
Executive offices: 740 Broadway, New York, New York 10003
Customer service and warehouse in care of:
Integrated Distribution Services,
195 McGregor St., Manchester, NH 03102, (603) 669-5933

Library of Congress Cataloging-in-Publication Data

Confronting life-threatening illness: Mind/body approaches.
   [Formerly titled: On the inside of illness]
   edited by Suzanne R. Engelman
      p. 295   cm. 15 x 23
   1. Medicine, Psychosomatic.
   I. Engelman, Suzanne R.
      [DNLM: 1. Disease–psychology. 2. Psychosomatic Medicine.
   3. Social Environment. QW 504 058]
   RC49.052   1993
   155.9'16–dc20
   DNLM/DLC
   for Library of Congress

90-4832
CIP

ISBN 0-8290-2473-5 (alk. paper)

First Printing 1993
1 3 5 7 9 10 8 6 4 2

Printed in the United States of America

Editor Credits

Suzanne R. Engelman, Ph.D. was formerly the Clinical Director at the Adult and Child Guidance Center, San Jose, California, and Assistant Clinical Professor with the Department of Psychiatry, University of California San Francisco Medical School, California. Dr. Engelman is the author of numerous articles in the fields of psychosomatics, health and the family, and humanistic psychology.

Dr. Engelman currently is in private practice in San Jose, California, where she lives with her husband and one year old son.

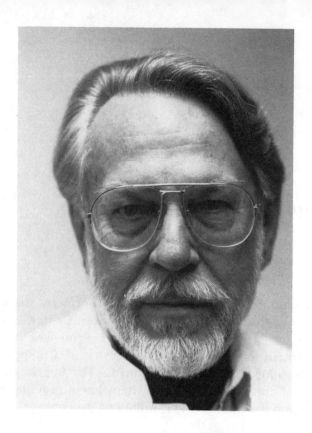

In Dedication:

Dr. Claus Bahne Bahnson is an unusual man in his wealth of talents; he is a pioneer researcher in the areas of psychosomatic influences in cancer, and has initiated critical investigations and conferences in that area. He is a sensitive clinician, finely tuned to psychological dynamic nuances and possessing a firm understanding of the inner dimensions of human relations. He is also a superb teacher and administrator in leading others in their scientific explorations. Dr. Bahnson's reputation is international—having been a leading figure in the American Academy of Psychoanalysis, International Psychosomatic Society, on the editorial boards of several scientific journals, and the author of over 130 articles and presentations (see Bahnson Bibliography in Appendix at back of book). Personally, Claus is a man of vision. His attributes of creativity in the arts, and a passion for life, present a man of unusual depth and character.

Dr. Bahnson is currently Professor of Psychiatry and Human Behavior at Jefferson Medical College, Thomas Jefferson University, Philadelphia; a member of the Board of Directors of John Rittmeister Institute, Kiel, Germany; Past President of the Nordic University, Flensburg, Germany; and Past Professor of Psychiatry (in Psychosomatics and Psychotherapy), University of California, San Francisco Medical School.

Dr. Bahnson may be reached by writing to him at Roon Strasse 3, D-2300 Kiel, Germany.

Table Of Contents

Preface .... *xi*
Dedication .... *xxi*
Introduction .... *xxv*

❖

Section I   *Evaluating Psychosocial Factors and Adaptation to Life-Threatening Illness*

Chapter 1   Annegret Boll, Ph.D.,
            Hubert Speidel, M.D.
            "Psychological and
            Social Rehabilitation after Heart Surgery" 3

Chapter 2   Atle Dyregrove, Ph.D.,
            Reidar Thyholdt, Ph.D.,
            Jeffrey T. Mitchell, Ph.D.
            "Rescue Worker's Emotional
            Reactions Following a Disaster" 31

Chapter 3 Wolfgang Jacob, M.D.
"The Sick Person in a Field of Tension
in Modern Society - Psychosis
and Carcinoma as a Counterpart" 46

Chapter 4 Margit von Kerekjarto, Ph.D.
"Considerations for the Impact of
Medical Therapy on Quality of Life" 56

❖

Section II Life-Threatening Illness: Mind-Body Approaches and Psychotherapy

Chapter 5 Rudolf Klussmann, M.D., and
Thomas Baumann, M.D.
"Working with AIDS-Patients" 68

Chapter 6 Thomas Küchler, Ph.D.
"Ethical Issues in Psychotherapy
With Cancer Patients" 85

Chapter 7 Hans Peter Bilek, M.D.
"Encouragement of the Incurably Ill" 94

Chapter 8 Suzanne R. Engelman, Ph.D.
"The Spiritual Dimensions of Working
With Families in a Medical Setting" 104

Chapter 9 Steven Fleck, M.D.
"The Family's Roles in Health
and Disease" 118

Chapter 10 Dan G. Hertz, M.D.
"On the Threshold of Death:
Implications of Impending Death
on Patients, Physicians and Families" 137

Section III Mind-Body Interactions and their Impact on Life-Threatening Illness

Chapter 11   Roger W. Bartrop, M.D., Ronald Penny, M.D., Lina Forcier, Ph.D., and Michael Jones "Grief, Immunity, and Morbidity: Psychophysiological Interactions" 158

Chapter 12   Dirk Fehlenberg, Ph.D., Karl Köhle, M.D. "Doctor-Patient Interaction During Daily Ward Rounds: The Traditional Setting and Exploration of the Psychosomatic Approach" 184

Chapter 13   Thure von Uexküll, M.D. "Psychosomatic Medicine and Aggression: Theoretical Considerations" 203

List of Contributors, Titles and Affiliations 225

List of Claus Bahne Bahnson's Reprints 227

Index
         Authors 243
         Subject 250

Preface

Norman Cousins

The fact that malignancies can be caused by emotional states is still regarded as a dubious proposition in some medical quarters but at least and at last there is a strong trend, backed by a substantial body of research, in the direction of recognizing that the mind interacts with the endocrine and immune systems in a way that can invite or combat serious disease. If lingering reluctance still exists in some quarters to accept the full implications of psychosocial factors in the cause and treatment of disease, imagine the situation as it was a quarter-century or more ago when Claus Bahne Bahnson first began to call attention to evidence showing that emotional stress could weaken the body's defenses against cancer. Bahnson was not merely a well-trained student of the workings of the human mind; he was a historian and philosopher of medicine as well. He connected the theories and findings of physicians over the centuries to current research on the biochemistry of the emotions. He reminded the profession that Galen, 2,000 years ago, observed a possible relationship between protracted melancholy and the onset of breast tumors. Claus undertook consistent and persistent studies of new research throughout the world bearing on the physiological effects of emotional strain. He drew together the strands of studies pointing to predictive factors, including data both on personality types that might be predisposed to serious illness and on life circumstances that figured in increased vulnerability or susceptibility.

Year by year, Claus has continued his tracking of new or extended research in the field, providing up-to-date reports and evaluations of the state of the art—all in addition, of course, to his own probes and insights. As a member of the UCLA Task Force on psychoneuroimmunology, he is a valuable resource for the entire group, with his relevant and significant correlations of thought and work being carried out elsewhere.

Bahnson's membership in the UCLA Task Force, in a very real sense, is an outgrowth of our own relationship going back to the early sixties. I had met him in connection with our mutual interest in world order as a prerequisite for a durable peace. It was in Copenhagen, I think, that representatives of the European Een Verden movement came together with representatives of the United World Federalists in a meeting of the World Association of World Federalists. Claus and I were able to get off by ourselves for part of the time and I became fascinated with the account of his studies in the area of mind/body relationships. Not long afterwards, Claus wrote an article for *The Saturday Review*, of which I was then editor, which introduced to a general American audience the then revolutionary concept that the emotions could have a role in exposing the body to cancer.

Claus continued to send me reprints of his subsequent contributions to medical journals. Consequently, after I joined the faculty of the UCLA School of Medicine, and was given the opportunity to develop the school's interest in the emerging field of psychoneuroimmunology, I lost no time in inviting Claus to become a regular member of our newly created task force. What made the connection possible was that Claus had then (1981) become a faculty member of the University of California, San Francisco, Medical School stationed at Fresno. He attended our meetings regularly and undertook research projects under the terms of a gift to the School of Medicine which I was asked to administer.

My own interest and involvement in the general area of mind/body studies was consistently encouraged by Claus. For some years I had been an admirer of Walter Cannon. His *Wisdom of the Body* led me to his other two major works—*Bodily Changes in Pain, Hunger, Fear and Rage,* and *The Way of an Investigator.* In turn, those books led to Cannon's student, Hans Selye, whose autobiography, *From Dream to Discovery,* struck me as a remarkable account of a superbly developed mind.

Cannon's writing also had the effect of leading me to the early pioneers of what was to become known much later as the field of psychoneuroimmunology. I learned about the work of Friedrich Bidder and Carl Schmidt, of Germany, who in 1852 observed the effects of emotional states on the digestive systems of animals. Cannon was a careful observer of the work of Pavlov, who is principally known for his findings on conditioned reflexes. But it is possibly that an even more significant contribution may be Pavlov's observations on the relationship between expectations and gastric changes in animals. Cannon gave the name "psychic secretions" to this effect. One of Cannon's most interesting observations was that, under circumstances of heightened emotion, the spleen could increase the red blood cell population by up to 30 percent.

Cannon had a well-balanced view of the entire field of mind/body studies. He was equally critical of pathologists who asked for hard morphological evidence showing that the mind had any effect on disease, and of mystics who overstated the role of the mind in healing. Both these groups, he said, needed an accurate understanding of the physiological processes which accompany profound emotional experiences. His substantial research identified a wide range of bodily disturbances caused by the emotions. *Bodily Changes in Pain, Hunger, Fear and Rage* summarized 42 papers by members of Harvard's physiological laboratory on the effects of emotion on the nervous system, the endocrine system, and the digestive system.

One of Cannon's contemporaries, Fritz Mohr, the noted German medical scientist, made a pithy summary of the matter when he observed that "there is no such thing as purely psychic illness or a purely physical one—only a living event taking place in a living organism which is itself alive only by virtue of the fact that in it psychic and somatic are united."

Among others who helped prepare the way for psychoneuroimmunology were medical researchers like Selye, Alexander, Meyer, Engel, Bernard, Wolf, Beecher, Menninger, Wyss, Reshauer, and Heyer, who had accumulated scientific evidence on the way the mind makes its registrations on human physiology. One of the most striking recent descriptions of the interaction is to be found in Lewis Thomas' description of wart removal by hypnosis in his book, *The Medusa and the Snail.* He observed that warts "can be made to go away by something that can only be called thinking, or something like thinking." He also pointed to the mysterious involvement of the immune system in this process, with the various classes of lymphocytes summoned to do their work. The phenomena served as the basis for our special studies at UCLA.

In describing our work to Claus, I told him that within a few months after coming to UCLA, I found myself in an unanticipated role. The announcement that I had been appointed to the medical faculty was interpreted by a segment of the public to mean that I was to serve as a medical ombudsman. I began to receive telephone calls or letters from people who had special problems or grievances—with the medical community in general rather than with the UCLA physicians in particular. The preponderance of these calls was concerned not with treatments or procedures but with the kinds of situations that had their origins in faulty patient-physician relationships.

> *Example:* A woman said she had undergone a series of diagnostic tests. The physician told her that he hadn't yet seen the results of the tests but he was "pretty sure it's cancer." The patient complained that the physician was being unscientific and unprofessional in his apparent haste to offer a terrifying speculation. (The tests turned out to be negative.)
>
> *Example:* The wife of a cancer patient complained that the physician in charge of the case came into her husband's hospital room and spoke to them from near

the doorway. There was no effort to ease the shock of what he had to say; he came flat out and said the tests were completed and that the news was "very bad." When asked just how bad, he said the diagnosis was cancer and that it was terminal. I asked the woman whether she preferred that the physician not tell the truth. She replied that she didn't object to being told the truth; what troubled her was the insensitive manner in which the truth was delivered.

Example: A woman complained that she waited almost two hours in the physician's waiting room for a report of a breast biopsy. Finally, she was brought into the physician's office and was informed that the biopsy was negative. As she was leaving, she was called back by the nurse and told there had been an unfortunate slip-up in the records and that the biopsy had been positive, after all. She asked to speak to the physician but was told that he was behind schedule and would be unable to see her.

Example: A patient, having gone through rigorous diagnostic procedures, asked the physician what he had found. "If I were you," the physician said, according to the patient, "I would get my affairs in order as quickly as possible." Again, it was the casual and inartistic method of communication that served as the basis for the grievance.

Example: A physician telephoned the patient, saying that the results of the tests were at hand and that it was imperative for her to check into the hospital immediately. He would meet her at the admissions desk in one hour. On arrival at the hospital, the woman learned that the physician had been called away. It was more than an hour before he returned, at which time it was discovered that there had been a mistake and that a room was not available after all. She was advised to go home and return the following morning. The patient complained that she had been scared out of her wits by the summons to the hospital and was bewildered by the casualness with which she was now told that it would be all right to come back the next day.

What most of these complaints had in common was that the patients felt they had not been treated with adequate respect or sensitivity. Next in order of magnitude were complaints about the size of the physician's bills. Some of these patients were on Medicare or medical insurance and therefore were not directly affected by the bills; they complained nonetheless that the government or the insurance companies were being made to pay stiff fees for a multitude of tests that might or might not have been necessary.

One woman (I attach no particular significance to the fact that ninety percent of the callers were women) said she didn't understand why she should have been put through a battery of exploratory tests costing several hundred dollars for what she had been told at the outset was an inflammation of her inner ear. In her indignation, she went to another physician who confirmed the original diagnosis in a matter of minutes. His bill was one-tenth that presented by the first physician.

A surprisingly large number of complaints were resolved to the satisfaction of the patients as the result of new discussions with the physicians involved. It developed that many of the patients had misunderstood the physicians or had misinterpreted the medical issues involved. I was struck with the frequency with which poor communication, rather than poor treatment, served as the basis for the complaints.

These observations were consistent with Claus' own writings, especially in his description of the impact of illness on the mind-set of patients.

Between June, 1978, when I began the association with UCLA, and August, 1987, I met with some 450 patients suffering from various forms of cancer. Nothing about these patients was more striking to me than that many of them experienced a sharp downturn in their condition coincident with the diagnosis. The moment they had an ominous label to attach to their symptoms, their condition worsened. At first, I thought these patients had delayed too long in seeing their physicians. This turned out to be true in a few cases; in most, what had happened was that the shock of the bad news became an intensifying factor.

Why should this be? Why should knowing what is wrong make one worse? Why should the diagnosis of an illness, in some cases, become a complicating factor in the treatment?

While I was pondering these questions, I saw a newspaper item that offered a possible clue. The item reported that ambulances from five hospitals had to ply back and forth between emergency rooms and a football stadium in Monterey Park, on the east side of Los Angeles, because of an imaginary epidemic of food poisoning. What had happened was that a half-dozen persons reported ill during the game. The examining physician was able to ascertain that all of them had consumed soft drinks from the dispensing machines under the stands. He considered the possibility that the syrup in the drink might have been contaminated. Also, the dispensing machines were connected to copper piping; had copper sulfate leaked into the beverages? In an effort to protect the spectators, school authorities ordered that an announcement be made over the loudspeaker requesting that no one patronize the dispensing machines because some persons had become ill with food poisoning.

The moment this announcement was made, the entire stadium became a sea of retching and fainting people. More than one hundred of them had to be hospitalized. Then it was ascertained that the soft drinks were entirely innocent and the word was passed along. The illnesses vanished as suddenly as they had appeared.

In both cases, the critical agent was language. Words were processed by the human mind in a way that made for illness or recovery. My focus sharpened on the way people reacted to a diagnosis. If people at a sports event could become sick enough to be hospitalized just as the result of an announcement over a loudspeaker, what would the effect be of a diagnosis of cancer, or, for that matter, of any life-threatening illness?

The phenomenon of mass psychogenic illness was hardly new. In the Middle Ages, many thousands of people throughout the European continent were seized by an imaginary disease that caused them to "dance" uncontrollably. At about the same time, thousands of people in Italy suffered from imaginary spider bites in what came to be known as the "tarantis epidemic." Jean Martin Charcot, Freud's teacher, furnished the scientific explanation in his ideas on "conversion hysteria."

Hardly less striking than the effects of a panic reaction to a serious diagnosis among the cancer patients I saw was the evidence that some patients had an opposite experience; that is, they had lived significantly longer than had been predicted by their oncologists. Almost two hundred of these survivors had come together in a group known as the "Wellness Community." They have a building or community center of their own in Santa Monica, California, provided by Harold Benjamin, an attorney and civic-minded citizen. These people have joined forces not just for the purpose of celebrating their longevity but to help meet the emotional needs of newly diagnosed cancer patients.

I met with some fifty or sixty members of this group at their center in an effort to learn how they themselves perceived the reasons for their extended longevity. One woman in her upper seventies—she had the kind of serene and beautiful features one associated with Grace Kelly—said she had a very clear idea of a turning point for the better in her own case. It came, she said, very early. The physician said he had the results of all the tests at hand, was making an unequivocal diagnosis of terminal cancer, and was giving her four to six months to live.

"I looked him straight in the eye," she said, "and told him to jump in the lake. That was six years ago."

Everyone cheered. Mrs. A. epitomized the experience of the group. They didn't deny the diagnosis; they denied the verdict that went with it. The denial took the form of a blazing determination and it was a window on the future. The range of their longevity beyond the predicted time ran from a half year to nine years. Most of them are still under treatment. They are able, many of them, to increase their tolerance of chemotherapy by subordinating their fears of it to their awareness that modern medical science is able to do war with cancers directly inside their bodies. They do not expect that the battle is without strain or sacrifice. But the important thing is that the battle is being joined and they are throwing all their resources into the fight.

I thought about these contrasting groups—those who panicked at the time of the diagnosis and experienced a downturn, and those who regarded the diagnosis as a challenge and who provided their physicians with an auspicious climate for treatment. I had no way of knowing whether I was correct in believing that the way the physician communicates has a bearing on the outcome of a case; I was dealing with subjective materials and not with scientific data. In discussing this possibility with my colleagues at the medical school, I recognized that physicians were right in asking for systematic, verifiable, and reproducible evidence. Also, they wanted proof that the patient's own approach to the illness could have clinical significance. How to develop such data? To what extent do depression and anxiety complicate an illness and impose an additional burden on treatment? Is it possible that liberating a patient from severe depression and anxiety may have significance in enhancing the prospects for effective treatment?

Claus Bahne Bahnson's work over the years has provided important leads to all these questions and has figured prominently in the approach of the UCLA Task Force on Psychoneuroimmunology in creating its own research projects. The most far-reaching of these projects perhaps has been examining the phenomena of depression and anxiety under circumstances of life-threatening illness. Several hundred cancer patients are involved in this research, divided according to types of cancer, with corresponding controls. All groups receive the required medical treatment. Members of the research group, however, also participate in special sessions in which they are educated about the nature of their particular illness, are put in touch with patients who have survived the same disease, are counseled in coping techniques, and are given simple biofeedback exercises for the purpose of demonstrating that human beings are not barred from some measure of supervision over their autonomic functions. Most important of all, perhaps, the members of the group interact with one another and are part of a collective experience designed to lift them out of feelings of depression, anxiety, loneliness, and alienation.

The project has been in existence for little more than a year. It will be at least another year before significant data will be available. It is not too early, however, to discern interesting trends indicated by the first 45 patients. Reduction of depression is marked by a proportionate increase in interleukins, which play a key role in the immune system. Equally significant so far is the evidence that reduction of depression does not depend exclusively on special psychological or educational techniques. It is apparent that medical treatment in which the patient feels a degree of involvement can have value in reducing depression and its effects. It may be significant that, even without special training or supervised activities, individuals who can be liberated from severe emotional strain during treatment enjoy enhanced prospects for effective medical care.

Even when this research is completed, it can only provide partial answers. However, together with studies being carried out at some dozen or more other centers under such investigators as Claus Bahne Bahnson, Robert Ader, George Engel, Novera Herbert Spector, Ronald Glaser, Kathleen Dillon, Karen Bulloch, Mark Laudenslager, Joan Borysenko, Joel Elkes, David McClelland, and others, it may be possible to identify some of the pathways and processes involved in the interaction between the nervous system, the endocrine system, and the immune system. Medical researchers, in the language of the Supreme Court, are proceeding with "deliberate speed," to develop evidence about mind/body connections—connections that have to be demonstrated and not assumed.

Claus Bahne Bahnson is one of the pioneers in this entire field. This book is a fitting tribute to a scientist, philosopher, educator, and most of all, a gifted comprehender of the human situation.

Dedication
Hommage à Claus

by Ebbe Linnemann

Perhaps the only real friend Van Gogh had was his brother Theo who, during Van Gogh's short span of life, was touching in his concern for his sick brother.

Theo was an art dealer in Paris, where he managed with great trouble to sell one of Vincent's paintings; one single painting during the whole of Vincent's life. They corresponded and their correspondence is something of a gold mine to an understanding of what happens in a sick but continuously creative mind.

Paul Gauguin once stayed with Van Gogh in Arles. They did not really like each other and would differ wildly about a great many things. Especially about the art of painting. They argued and in the middle of one of their arguments Van Gogh cut off his ear. Paul Gauguin was horrified and fled headlong. Van Gogh was then admitted to a mental hospital.

From the hospital he wrote to Theo: "Even if a lot of people in this hospital are very ill, I feel as if the fear and terror I used to have for insanity, has weakened. And even though I constantly hear terrible screams like from animals in a menagerie, people here are friendly and help each other when in crises. When I am working in the garden they all come and watch, and I can assure you they are more considerate and polite than the good citizens of Arles." Van Gogh was admitted to a mental hospital several times and it did him good. Owing to this was not the least that one of the doctors took great care of him and allowed him much freedom to paint. Some of his most beautiful paintings derive from his stay in the hospital.

It is obvious from his correspondence that it was a tremendous relief to him to be admitted to the hospital, when he was tormented by delusions. This is an aspect in the functioning of a mental hospital we today are apt to overlook.

The gifted Norwegian author Jens Bjorneboe took his own life in 1976. He was an alcoholic and at times insane. "Obviously I suffer from all known forms of alcoholism. I am a true dipsomaniac. I drink in periods and I drink every day. I drink from habit. I drink socially and occasionally, but I most certainly also drink when alone," he writes about himself, not without a sense of humor. Somewhere else he writes: "What would largely have become of our lovely, beautiful, stinking Europe without our drug addicts, alcoholics, the sexual minorities, the T.B. sufferers, the mental cases, the syphilitics, those who suffer from nocturnal enuresis (bedwetters), the criminals, the epileptics? Our whole civilization is created by criminals and mental cases. A normal person who has done any useful thing does not exist. Those who built slave-labor camps in Russia and Germany were normal people."

Dostoevsky was an epileptic. Few like him have a depth of insight into human mind. In one of his novels he writes: "Every human being keeps in his memory thoughts which cannot be admitted to everyone, perhaps only to friends. Besides, there are also thoughts which cannot even be admitted to friends; only to oneself and in deep secrecy. Finally there are thoughts man would not even admit to himself. In every well organized human being there exists a considerable amount of such thoughts and the more rigid a person is the more inhibited." It is not hard to understand that Freud learned a lot by reading Dostoevsky.

All these haphazardly chosen artists (and a lot of others might have been mentioned) have something in common: the urge to create new life, always to go on and never stopping to breathe. All this they have in common with Claus Bahne Bahnson who is also an artist. Like them he has never been afraid to take new steps, to open up new dimensions to us. But he is at the same time also a scientist who has never abandoned himself to emotional blindness and has always been capable of purifying his anxiety with his bright intellect. This continuous, painful tension, this ceaseless inner dialogue has made Claus such a fine psychotherapist.

Like his countryman Soren Kierkegaard, he can with a clear conscience, demand from the person who wants to call himself a helper to human beings:

> That if real success is to attend the effort to bring a man to a definite position, one must first of all take pains to find HIM where he is and begin there.
>
> This is the secret of the art of helping others. Anyone who has not mastered this is himself deluded when he proposes to help others. In order to help another effectively I must understand more than he—yet first of all surely I must understand what he understands. If I do not know that, my greater understanding will be of no help to him. If, however, I am disposed to plume myself on my greater understanding, it is because I am vain or proud, so that at bottom, instead of benefiting him, I want to be admired. But all true effort to help begins with self-humiliation: the helper must first humble himself and therewith must understand that to help does not mean to be ambitious but to be patient, that to help means to endure for the time being the imputation that one is in the wrong and does not understand what the other understands.
>
> Take the case of a man who is passionately angry, and let us assume that he is really in the wrong. Unless you can begin with him by making it seem as if it were he that had to instruct you, and unless you can do it in

such a way that the angry man, who was too impatient to listen to a word of yours, is glad to discover in you a complaisant and attentive listener—if you cannot do that, you cannot help him at all.

Introduction

This volume entitled *Confronting Life-Threatening Illness: Mind-Body Approaches* consists of the works of researchers and clinicians in the fields of psychosomatics, mind-body interactions, and humanistic medicine. The inclusion in this volume of scientists from both Europe and the United States underscores the importance of the world community learning from one another's thinking to collectively advance our knowledge of health and illness.

Section I identifies and quantifies psychosocial factors affecting adaptation to life-threatening illness; Section II presents mind-body approaches used in the psychotherapy process of people with life-threatening illnesses and their families, including cancer, spinal-cord injury, heart disease, and AIDS. Section III delves into psychophysiological interactions and how they impact life-threatening illness. The immune system and other biologic components in interaction with the psyche are explored. Taken as a whole, this book represents a system's perspective of health and illness. This model recognizes the important interrelationships of the immune system, mind (including unconscious, and conscious communications), body, and environment (including the family, physician, and medical setting) as critically impacting health and illness.

The assistance of a large number of persons has made the completion of this volume possible. I would like to take this opportunity to recognize these individuals.

First, I would like to acknowledge the contributors who have spent many hours writing and revising their manuscripts. They have dedicated their manuscripts to honor Claus Bahne Bahnson for his pioneering work in studying the biopsychosocial interactions in health and illness. All of these scientists have helped to further our understanding of these important dimensions involved in the processes of healing and dying.

Second, I would like to thank Ms. Linda Weiss Bahnson for her time initially reviewing the manuscripts and serving as a consultant in the publication of *Confronting Life-Threatening Illness: Mind-Body Approaches*.

I also want to thank Dorothy Adams Montgomery for her fine typing skills, and for providing much good advice in the preparation of the volume.

Finally, I want to thank my husband, Dennis, whose love, support and interest have been much appreciated through the lengthy process of completing *Confronting Life-Threatening Illness: Mind-Body Approaches*.

Suzanne R. Engelman, Ph.D.
Editor, *Confronting Life-Threatening Illness: Mind-Body Approaches*.
San Jose, California

Section I
❖
Evaluating Psychosocial Factors and Adaptation to Life-Threatening Illness

1

Psychological and Social Rehabilitation after Heart Surgery

Annegret Boll, Hubert Speidel

Introduction

Claus Bahne Bahnson's studies on heart attacks (Bahnson & Wardwell, 1962) still rank among the best work on the psychosomatic aspects of the heart and circulation system; they have often been quoted and so far have not been bettered. His work can also serve as a useful guideline for research into another related field which has grown up since the mid 'fifties: heart surgery, and the specific effects it has on the patient.

From the very beginning it was apparent that a high rate of psychological disturbances could be expected during the first few days after such an operation, especially if extra-corporal circulation was involved. Even though the mortality rate has in the meantime sunk from the initial 20%-30% to below 5% and even to considerably below 1% for some types of heart operation, the psychological upheaval involved has become more and more obvious. Normally there is a "post-operative illness" (Speidel & Rodewald, 1980) on the second and third days after the operation, involving dramatic alterations in all the physiological parameters which sometimes reach pathological levels; the panic experienced by a delirious or psychotic patient can endanger the whole precarious metabolism because of the sudden demand for more oxygen, which can lead to a total collapse. Some heart surgeons, including for instance G. Rodewald in Hamburg (Rodewald, Kalmar & Krebber, 1982), paid particular attention to these aspects right from the outset, and sought the cooperation of psychiatrists and psychotherapists when treating his patients.

Interest was focused initially on listing and classifying these post-operative difficulties. Because there were no commonly agreed methods or schemes available for classifying them, the results were extremely contradictory (Speidel, Dahme, Flemming, Götze, Huse-Kleinstoll, Meffert, Rodewald & Spehr, 1978); the psychiatric morbidity rate, for instance, varied between 3% and 100% (Spiedel et al., 1978; Götze, Dahme & Wessel, 1980). The most thorough investigations showed that between 40% and 50% of the patients suffered from post-operative psychopathological disturbances. Attempts to classify these according to clinical criteria, which in themselves were highly varied, and then to analyze them along factor or cluster lines, proved highly confusing (Dahme, Flemming, Götze, Huse-Kleinstoll, Meffert & Speidel, 1982).

To remedy this situation and to enlist the help of the various research groups in Europe and the USA, our Hamburg study group organized an international symposium, to which we invited all the groups we knew. This symposium in 1978 (Speidel & Rodewald, 1980) was followed by a second one in Milwaukee (Becker, Katz, Polonius & Speidel, 1982), which led to a common research project and culminated in the foundation of an International Consortium for the Study of Neurological and Psychological Reactions to Cardiac Surgery. Its members worked out a set of categories which were translated into the various languages; since then they have been used in about a dozen centers in South, Central and North America and in various European countries and published as an International Study (for the study) of Neurological and Psychological Reactions to Cardiac Surgery.

While this ambitious project, which concentrated on the early post-operative disturbances after heart operations, was getting under way, interest began to focus not just on the periods shortly before and after the operation but on the years afterwards, and the problems the patients had to face in their private and public lives, briefly and inadequately termed "rehabilitation." It soon became clear that there was a great discrepancy between the rapid advances made in heart surgery, thanks to enormous investments in terms of money and skill, of which the surgeons could be justifiably proud, and the on-the-whole disappointing results if the emotional and social implications for the patients following the operation were taken into consideration (see also, Becker et al., 1982; Walter, 1985). We were forced to acknowledge that in this, as in other illnesses, the extent of the physical damage and the dysfunction resulting from it were not in themselves sufficient to enable us to prognose the possible subsequent psychological and social disadvantages for the patient. We began to regard the recovery process and its outcome as a phenomenon made up of many different facets (Waltz, 1981). How the patient adjusts medically, privately and professionally, emotionally and psychosomatically, each have to be examined separately and in relation to one another before we can say how successful the recovery has been.

Current State of Research

It is striking that the psychosomatic follow-ups of patients after heart surgery which have so far been carried out have made use of widely different methods. Generally speaking, however, the results available suggest that a relatively large proportion of patients still face considerable psychological and social difficulties a year or more after the operation (Boll, 1986). Heller and co-workers (1974) came to the conclusion that long-term rehabilitation in 39% of the patients did not measure up to the results of the operation; the recovery of these patients was hindered by emotional problems; in 21% of them the recovery process had to be regarded as severely impeded. Kimball (1976) stated that at least 20% of the patients would require either psychotherapeutic or psychiatric help during the course of their convalescence. After rating a psychoanalytic interview, Speidel and co-workers (1980) came to a total of 57% who needed psychotherapeutic help.

As far as the patients' subjective satisfaction with the results of the operation goes, Reimer and his co-workers (1982) noted there was a difference between patients who had undergone coronary artery bypass surgery (CABS) and those who had had a heart valve correction; roughly two-thirds of the latter were content with the result, whereas only a quarter of the patients with CABS were satisfied. G. Dahme, B. Dahme, Kornemann, Vollerts and Huse-Kleinstoll (1980), investigating the relationship between fulfilled and unfulfilled expectations about the operation, worked out a complex scale termed the index for subjective rehabilitation. 29% were rated as "poorly rehabilitated"; most of their expectations had not been fulfilled. The severity of the preoperative heart disease proved to be a significant factor for the prognosis.

When the patients were asked to make their own assessment of changes in their emotional well-being, about 50% of them reported that their mood improved as time went on; between 10% and 20% reported a change for the worse (Ross, Diwell, Marsh, Monro & Barker, 1978; Stanton, Zyzanski, Jenkins & Klein, 1982; Heller, Frank, Kornfeld, Wilson & Malm, 1982; Brown & Rawlinson, 1975).

Many of the long-term emotional and social problems which make matters worse for the patients were linked with employment problems. In both the USA and the Federal Republic of Germany, a large proportion of patients who have been employed before the operation are unemployed after it (Boll, 1986). In a survey (Speidel et al., 1981), we discovered that 20% of the patients did not return to work after the operation, and only 40% were fully rehabilitated. About half of those employed complained about having problems at work, and about a quarter of the patients on a disablement pension could not come to terms with their new status. In a sample of heart surgery patients who were pensioned off, Davies-Osterkamp and co-workers (1982) did not, however, come across a "pensioned-off syndrome" comparable with the depressive symptoms, such as a pronounced tendency to withdraw from social contacts and more psychosomatic complaints after becoming unemployed, as described by Johnson (1958). Financial difficulties seem to be more prevalent in the USA where there is no social security net comparable with that in West Germany; Stanton and others (1982) report that 30% of the patients had to contend with a reduction in income, whereas Speidel et al. (1981) report on only 15% who found it difficult to make ends meet.

If one looks at the state of the whole family in relation to the operation, the evidence from questionnaires shows that the situation generally improved after the operation (Ross et al., 1978; Brown & Rawlinson, 1979; Heller et al., 1982). In a survey of 67 patients, using an interview which included questions not immediately linked to the illness, we discovered that 36% felt their relationship to their partner was unsatisfactory, and 24% complained of tensions within the family (Speidel et al., 1981). Huse-Kleinstoll, Boll, Dahme, Götze, Meffert, Priebe & Speidel (1984a) have pointed out how important a happy partnership and support from the family are in helping the patient to cope with the psychological stress of being in the intensive care unit. Dahme et al. (1980) showed that the patient's rehabilitation was very much influenced by the attitudes of the spouse. There is often a close link between the difficulties within the partnership and sexual problems; in an interview more than a third of the patients reported sexual dysfunction, which they saw as linked to the operation and the illness. The proportion of patients who actually suffer from the dysfunction is, however, considerably lower; generally the failure to function sexually is regarded as inevitable or a sign of aging (Speidel, Boll, Dahme & Götze, 1985).

Long after the operation, patients continue to suffer from various kinds of psychopathological problems; in particular, they find it hard to concentrate and to remember. Götze and co-workers (1982) diagnosed a psycho-organic syndrome in about a quarter of the patients, a figure which Rabiner & Willner confirm (1980) in patients after heart valve replacement; in coronary patients, their figure was lower.

Studies on the course of recovery using standardized

personality tests have shown that a year after heart valve replacement the patients have less self-confidence than they had before the operation; they are less sociable and became more passive and withdrawn, they have less sexual appetite and rarely show any signs of displeasure or anger. Positive changes include an increased sense of responsibility in looking after themselves and a decrease in anxiety and dependency (Heller, Frank, Kornfeld, Malm & Bowman, 1974). Post-operatively, both patients with coronary disease and patients with heart valve defects show in the MMPI a markedly higher level of the "neurotic trio": hypochondria, hysteria and depression (Lutzenkirchen, Lamprecht, Walter & Dietz, 1980; Brown & Rawlinson, 1979).

Möhlen and co-workers (1982) examined to what extent the patient's long-term adjustment was influenced by the way he had coped with the prospect of having the operation; their results underline the importance of intact and stable ego functions and in particular of reliable defense mechanisms. Those patients who were able to retreat and concentrate on their own needs before the operation showed fewest depressive symptoms a year after it. Kimball and co-workers (1969) also saw a connection between pre-operative coping patterns and post-operative emotional stability. The patients who adapted to both illness and operation in a realistic and appropriate manner recovered more quickly; on the other hand strong symbiotic tendencies, pronounced denial of anxiety and marked depressive symptoms proved an unfavorable starting point.

Aims

The main purpose of this inquiry was to discover how well patients who have undergone heart surgery have adapted emotionally in the course of the three to five years which have elapsed since the operation. In particular, we sought answers to the following questions:

1. How well are the patients adjusted at the moment, and what differences are noticeable among them?

2. What links are there between the patients' long-term emotional adjustment and their mental, psychosocial, and professional rehabilitation?
3. What influence do preoperative psychological, social and somatic factors have on their long-term emotional well-being?
4. What emotional and psychosomatic changes do the patients notice, comparing how they felt just before the operation, 3-4 weeks after it and 3-5 years later?

Methods

Our sample consisted of 62 patients, 41 men (66%) and 21 women (34%). These patients are all part of a bigger sample which is being extensively scrutinized in an interdisciplinary research project, originally focusing on the psychopathological disturbances which became evident right after the operation, and the reasons for these. The average age of the patients when examined 3-5 years after the operation was 51-1/2 years. 34 patients (54%) had had a valve replacement, in 9 patients (15%) a congenital defect had been corrected, and 19 patients (31%) had had a CABS, with an additional aneurysmectomy where necessary.

At the time of this investigation 26 patients (42%) were holding down jobs, 30 patients (48%) were drawing pensions, 6 women patients were housewives without any supplementary pension. 12 patients (19%) retired after the operation, 18 patients (29%) had already retired before it.

These patients were examined before the operation and several times after it (1st-4th post-operative day interval, 7th-10th post-operative day interval, 3rd-4th post-operative week interval, 3rd-5th post-operative year interval) by means of a battery of tests. The psychological and psychiatric data were obtained through a combination of objective and subjective assessments, and used to establish both cross-section and long-term diagnosis. The customary personality tests and methods of rating, such as the Freiburger Personality Inventory (FPI) (Fahrenberg, Selg & Hampel, 1978), the Saarbruecken Anxiety List (SAL) (Spreen, 1961), the Giessen Test (GT) (Beckmann & Richter, 1972), the complaint list (von Kerekjarto, Meyer & von Zerssen, 1972) and Cohen's polarity profile (Cohen, 1969) were augmented by mood lists, and questionnaire and interviews designed by ourselves for this specific situation (Boll, 1986). Psychopathological disturbances were established by means of the AMDP, which is available in an abbreviated form in English (HRPD) (Götze et al., 1985).

Results

The variables which show how the patients adapted 3-5 years after the operation are those usually examined when inquiring into the psychosomatic aspects of chronic disease: the severity and frequency of depressive moods and anxiety, the incidence of psychosomatic complaints and the way the patient relates to others (Adams & Lindemann, 1974; Lipowsky, 1977; Sakinofsky, 1980; Joraschky & Köhle, 1981; Waltz, 1981). The personality tests used were SAL, "Basic Mood" scale from the GT, "Psychosomatic Disturbances" scale from the FPI, "Social Resonance" scale from the GT.

Our aim was to find groups of patients who adapted psychologically in a similar manner i.e., to discover a multidimensional criterion for successful long-term psychological adjustment. To do this the data from the variables were subjected to cluster analysis (interactive k-Means cluster analysis) (Spaeth, 1975). The result was four clusters (see Figure 1) which are statistically adequate and psychologically plausible; their validity was checked by comparing the 3- and 5-cluster solution and by a random alteration in the size of the sample.

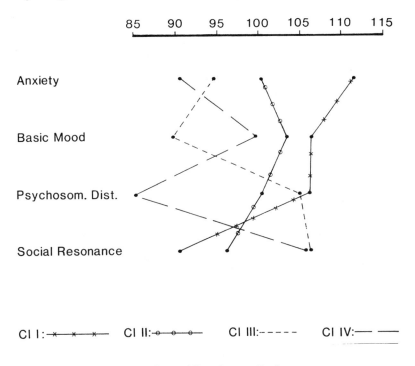

Figure 1. Profiles of the four criterion groups

The clusters were named as follows, in line with the profile values:

Group I (Labile) consists of 13 patients (21%) with considerable emotional and vegetative instability and a feeling of lack of positive social resonance.

Group II (Moderate) consists of 20 patients (32%) who had moderate levels in all four variables.

Group III (Psychosomatically disturbed) consists of 16 patients (26%) who are emotionally stable and have high positive social resonance; the level of psychosomatic problems compared with the other variables is high.

Group IV (Stable) consists of 13 patients (21%) who are emotionally and physically stable and have a high positive social resonance.

There are no differences between these four groups as far as age, sex or somatic diagnosis were concerned.

The validity of this grouping is underlined by significant differences in ratings of the patients' emotional strain reached by means of a psychoanalytically-oriented interview (see Tables 1 and 2).

Table 1
Comparison Between the Four Groups:
Incidence of Negative Emotional Changes

	Cluster				
	I	II	III	IV	
No	4	8	13	7	32
Yes	8	11	3	5	27
Total	12	19	16	12	59

$CHI^2 = 8.02$; df = 3; p = .05

Table 2 covers the distribution of patients with/without problems connected with death and dying.

Table 2
Comparison Between the Four Groups:
Incidence of Problems Connected With Death and Dying

	Cluster				
	I	II	III	IV	
No	4	15	13	7	39
Yes	8	4	3	5	20
Total	12	19	16	12	59

$CHI^2 = 9.11$; df = 3; p = .03

As might be expected, the emotionally unstable patients from Cluster I (Labile) have most problems in this sphere: two-thirds of the patients report increased emotional problems and are troubled by thinking about death. Cluster II is particularly interesting: these are the patients who have moderate values in all four variables when describing their own state of mind. A relatively high proportion (11 out of 19) reported an increase in emotional suffering. Only four of them, however, complained that the increased emotional strain was connected with death and dying. The patients in Cluster III (Psychosomatically disturbed) reported least suffering; only a quarter of them noticed a change for the worse in both areas. About half the patients in Cluster IV (Stable) complained of increased emotional suffering and problems connected with death and dying. This result is surprising if one compares it with the levels obtained from their own assessment of their mental state, which suggested that they are persons with a high emotional stability.

Table 3 shows the differences in the diagnosis of psychopathological symptoms (AMDP) among the four groups.

Table 3
Comparison Between the Four Groups: Type and Incidence of Psychopathological Symptoms at the Time of the Follow-Up

	Cluster				
	I	II	III	IV	
Free of symptoms	3	8	11	11	33
Slight psycho-organic syndrome	2	2	0	0	4
Phobic-hypochondriac	6	8	2	1	17
Affective-emotional syndrome with psycho-organic disturbances	2	2	3	1	8
Total	13	20	16	13	62

$CHI^2 = 16.73$; $df = 9$; $p = .05$

It is worth noting that with three exceptions the patients who were free of symptoms are to be found in Clusters II, III and IV. Taking the psychopathological symptoms as a whole, the four groups can be reorganized into two larger units: Clusters I (Labile) and II (Moderate) contained most (75%) of the patients with psychopathological symptoms. Those patients with psycho-organic disturbances, phobic-hypochondriac attitudes and emotional disturbances linked with impaired mental functioning are distributed more or less evenly in these two clusters. There are proportionally more patients free of symptoms in Cluster II (8 out of 20).

Medical Rehabilitation

Both the objective somatic condition of the patients and their subjective state of health were taken into account to find out to what extent the patients recovered physically (Lempp, 1983). We found clearly significant and possibly significant differences in the patients' subjective assessments of the severity of their stenocardia, psychosomatic complaints and cardiac arrhythmias. The objective findings did not reveal any differences between the groups except for cardiac arrhythmias. The patients in Cluster I and to a lesser extent in Cluster II judged their state of health to be worse than the patients in Clusters III and IV.

If one compares the objective cardiac findings with the subjective complaints, it is obvious that in all four clusters, the complaints seem subjectively more serious than the objective findings would seem to merit; the highest discrepancy can be found in Cluster I. This point can best be illustrated by the cardiac arrhythmias:

Table 4
Comparison Between the Four Groups: Objective Findings on the Severity of the Cardiac Arrhythmias

	Cluster				
	I	II	III	IV	
No cardiac arrhythmias	10	11	5	6	32
Occasional extra-systoli	0	6	7	4	17
Frequent or multi-focal extra-systoli	2	1	4	2	9
Total	12	18	16	12	58

$CHI^2 = 10.48$; df = 6; p = .1

Table 5
Comparison Between the Four Groups: Subjective Assessment of Severity of Cardiac Arrhythmias

	Cluster				
	I	II	III	IV	
No complaints	0	5	1	4	10
Moderate complaints	8	8	13	8	37
Severe complaints	4	5	2	0	11
Total	12	18	16	12	58

$CHI^2 = 12.67$; df = 6; p = .048

It is worth noting that a relatively high proportion of patients (4 out of 16) in Cluster III (Psychosomatically disturbed) have frequent or multifocal extra-systoli. Occasional extra-systoli were diagnosed in a further seven patients; in all, extra-systoli were observed in 70% of the patients. In contrast, only two out of 10 (20%) patients in Cluster I have extra-systoli, in Cluster II 40%, and in Cluster IV 50%.

As far as the patients' subjective assessment of the severity of their cardiac arrhythmias is concerned (Table 5), all the patients in Cluster I complain of having signs of them, although in fact only two patients were diagnosed as having them.

The same applies to a lesser extent to the other clusters: The rate of subjective complaints is higher than might be anticipated from the objective findings. Cluster IV (Stable) is the only group in which none of the patients suffer from severe complaints, although two of them have frequent or multifocal extra-systoli. Almost all the patients in Cluster III (15 out of 16) reported feeling affected by subjectively experienced cardiac arrhythmias.

Professional and Social Rehabilitation

Those patients who are now more or less reintegrated in professional life are equally distributed among the four clusters. We did not discover any "pensioned-off syndrome." The financial situation, however, does make a difference; there is a clear link with psychological adjustment. Of the nine patients who reported having financial problems, five come from Cluster I (Labile).

We did not find any statistically significant relationship between the family problems or the partnership problems and our criterion. There is, however, a correlation between marital and financial problems, which suggests that these two areas of conflict are closely interlinked.

Prognosis of Long-Term Psychological Adjustment

Altogether we looked into 22 different variables associated with the patient's state of mind, his psychosocial situation and his characteristic responses to the operation; these were measured just before the operation and during the 7th-10th day interval after it. Only three variables proved to have any lasting influence on the patient's long-term psychological adjustment: the preoperative diagnosis of a dominant personality, negative emotional changes brought on by the illness, and the post-operative assessment of passivity (see Table 6).

Table 6
Results of the Analysis of Variance of Mean Differences Between the Four Groups: Pre- and Post-Operative Psychological Factors

Variable	Cluster I	II	III	IV	F	p
Dominance	23.23	20.79	25.3	25.5	3.69	.02
Negative emotional-changes	38.00	32.67	34.75	29.67	2.33	.09
Passivity	22.08	25.37	22.00	22.73	2.67	.06

The difference in the preoperative assessment of dominance means that patients who 3-5 years later show low anxiety and depression and have considerable positive social resonance, were assessed before the operation as more dominant. The patients in Cluster I who show high negative ratings in all variables were preoperatively noticeable for their recurrent and powerful emotional reactions under the stress of the illness. These patients did, however, also tend to be more seriously ill; the preoperatively diagnosed level of heart insufficiency is higher in this group than in Clusters II and IV, but lower than in Cluster III (Table 7).

Table 7
Mean Differences Between the Four Groups: Preoperative Heart Insufficiency

	Cluster					
Variable	I	II	III	IV	F	p
State of heart insufficiency (NYHA)	2.95	2.68	3.13	2.62	2.34	.08

We should like to stress that the type and severity of the operation itself have no influence on the patients' subsequent psychological adjustment 3-5 years later. Similarly, the initial post-operative psychopathological disturbances, which were often dramatic and appeared in the guise of glittering symptoms, proved to be irrelevant as far as the long-term emotional prognosis is concerned. The same applies to the preoperative psychopathological disturbances.

Longitudinal Comparisons

In order to make longitudinal comparisons, we used the 12 scales of the FPI and the SAL, four scales of a multidimensional mood questionnaire and the complaint list on three separate occasions: before the operation, in the 3rd-4th post-operative week and 3-5 years after the operation. By using 2-factor analysis of variance, we could differentiate effects of grouping, time and their interaction.

16 of the 20 features examined revealed a significant time effect when analyzed in this manner. It is typical for these variables that the mean values after the operation (3rd to 4th week) contain least evidence of neurotic tendencies. After 3-5 years the mean values for emotional and vegetative instability have again reached the preoperative level or even exceed it; this is the case for manifest anxiety and the sum total of physical and emotional complaints reported by the patient. To illustrate this typical change over the course of time, here is a graph

showing how the variable "manifest anxiety" alters in the various groups.

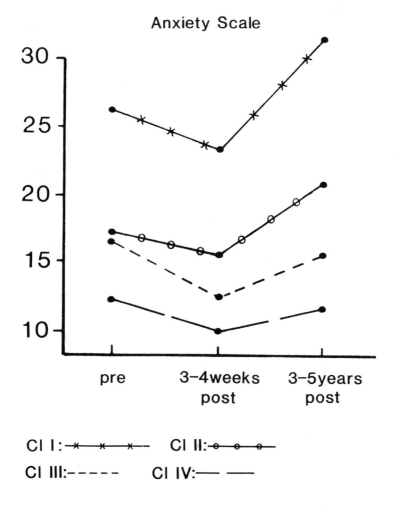

Figure 2. The course of anxiety datas over time

While all the patients show a general tendency to develop over the course of time, the more interesting point is the question of how the four groups alter differently over this period. Analysis of variance confirmed the following significant changes: psychosomatic disturbances (FPI), initiative and activeness (mood list), total number of complaints, feeling weak and short of breath (list of complaints). Figure 3 shows the trends for the changes in the four groups taking the total number of complaints as an example. This variable can be regarded as a general gauge of the patient's tendency to complain, either about psychic or about physical symptoms.

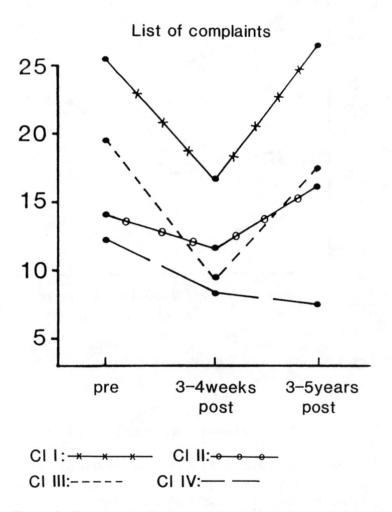

Figure 3. The course of complaintiveness datas over time

The patients in Cluster I tend to complain more about emotional, psychosomatic and physical (especially cardiac) symptoms and feel less and less active as time goes on. It looks as though the labile patients in Cluster I are far more fixated on their bodies and hearts than the other patients.

Taking into account the somatic results gained 3-5 years after the operation, we can conclude that the intensified interest in the body cannot be judged as an appropriate psychic reaction in regard to a worrying, life-threatening physical condition. The above-average increase in emotional and physical complaints in this patient group occurs in the period between hospital discharge and the time of the follow-up.

The patients of Cluster III characterized by their relatively high rate of psychosomatic disturbances, show a disproportionatelly high increase in complaints from the preoperative to the catamnestic point of time. In the same period the rate of complaints decreases with the stable patients of Cluster IV.

Discussion

Two main lines of inquiry have emerged in research into psychic disturbances after heart surgery: comparing the findings made under comparable conditions in different heart centers, and looking into the subsequent effects on the patients' states of mind and how to predict these. In our previous studies we tried to identify the psychosocial risk factors which affect the patients' emotional and mental adaptation to the illness and their reintegration into professional life. In this study we tried, with empirical backing, to describe the personality which is at risk.

By using cluster analysis, an empirical-statistical method, we were able to identify four clusters or groups of patients 3-5 years after the operation who adapted in different ways to heart surgery and chronic heart disease. These groups differed in the following ways: the extent to which the patients are anxious and depressed, the number of psychosomatic disturbances which affects them, and the quality of their social resonance. The groups include Group I, which on account of its high level of emotional and vegetative instability and its feeling of negative social resonance can be termed "Labile"; Group II, the so-called "Moderate" group; Group III, which is only remarkable for its high incidence of psychosomatic disturbances; and Group IV, whose test values suggest a high level of emotional and vegetative stability and positive social resonance.

While Brown and Rawlinson (1979), Lützenkirchen et al. (1980) and Heller et al. (1982) in their follow-ups could detect general trends which were valid for the entire sample when comparing them with either the preoperative level or the normal population, our results gained by cluster analysis answer the question: In which and how many patients are distress reactions greater or smaller than expected? 21% of our sample (Group I) show clear signs of above-average emotional, physical and social distress. This proportion tallies with the findings made by Heller et al. (1974), Kimball (1976) and Dahme et al. (1980), who also identified at least 20% of the patients after heart surgery as having serious long-term psychological problems which called for psychiatric or psychotherapeutic help.

Emotional strain, especially in the form of experienced and verbalized anxiety, is the result of a complex interplay between the type and intensity of the anxiety stimuli and the patient's more or less stable defenses against them (Huse-Kleinstoll et al., 1984b). Among the sources of anxiety for patients after heart operations are, apart from intrapsychic neurotic fears, above all the burden of being chronically ill and facing the prospect of a deterioration, coupled with problems linked with the patient's social environment, such as uncertainties about returning to work or financial difficulties. Whether the defense mechanisms can cope with such anxieties, depends on the quality of the patient's ego-functions; any impairment due to reduced mental functioning, as revealed when the patient has difficulties in paying attention, concentrating or remembering, or due to severe pain, can make the task of coping much more difficult.

Looking at our results one can say, generally speaking, that at the time of the follow-up the coping abilities of the anxious and depressive patients with their weakened defense mechanisms are additionally severely hindered by psychopathological disturbances. These patients also have more psychosocial problems, especially connected with money. However, objectively measuring, they are not more seriously ill than the other patients; i.e., going by the medical findings, heart disease does not pose a greater threat to these patients than to the others, contrary to what one might have supposed.

While the levels reported by Group IV (Stable) when describing their own condition suggest that they have consistently stable defenses, their resistance proved more vulnerable when they were interviewed. The fact that almost half the patients in this group admitted to worrying about death and dying, could be taken as a hint at some buried intrapsychic conflict which is kept fairly well repressed; the interviewer's presence and understanding made it possible for the patients to admit this.

From the small number of negative emotional changes or problems associated with death and dying found in Cluster III (Psychosomatically disturbed), we can conclude that the tendency to somatize, which is demonstrated by the higher rate of physical complaints, acts as a relatively stable form of defense.

One central issue is the long-term correlation between the degree of medical rehabilitation and psychological adjustment in chronically ill patients. Our results suggest there is little connection between the objective medical findings and the patient's state of mind; on the other hand there is a clear correlation between the psychological findings and the subjective cardiac complaints caused by cardiac arrhythmias and stenocardia.

The severity of such complaints is more pronounced in Group I and, to a lesser extent, also in Group II than might have been expected from the objective findings, so that one gets the impression that these patients are hyperconscious of their hearts, and that their basically anxious and depressive attitude has hypochondriacal elements. We found no justification whatsoever for the assumption that the labile patients in Cluster I are more severely, or even fatally ill, as might have been concluded from the distress they experience subjectively.

The danger that a particular patient will have difficulties in adjusting to the operation and its consequences can be prognosed before the operation. Considerable habitual emotional and vegetative instability before the operation, coupled with a great deal of strain arising from the heart disease which the patient can barely cope with, plus a pronounced heart insufficiency and a non-dominant, passive and dependent attitude are all serious risk factors for the patient's successful rehabilitation 3-5 years later. These results confirm the importance of preoperatively intact ego functions, postulated by Möhlen and co-workers (1982), and the negative prognostic significance of regressive, symbiotic tendencies before the operation (Kimball, 1969; Heller et al., 1974). Unusually powerful emotional reactions to stress before the operation brought about by the disease itself, as seen in the labile patients in Group I, can be interpreted as a sign that this group could not cope adequately with the burden and strains inherent in this disease even before the operation. This means that such patients undergo surgery in a state when their defenses are already shaky, and that they do not have the resources to protect themselves from the anxiety, insecurity and resignation which the operation and the post-operative course induce in them. Huse-Kleinstoll et al. (1984a) have already identified a high level of emotional stress caused by the illness itself as a risk factor when the patient is confronted with the pressures involved in a stay in the intensive care unit.

The observation that the four groups change in different ways psychologically and somatically as time passes provides us with a new detail to fill out our picture of the recovery process. It is not just the patient's preoperative psychological and psychosomatic condition which determines how the patients in Cluster I fare subsequently; after the operation these patients clearly show negative deviations from the rest of the sample, especially concerning the number of emotional and physical complaints they report.

If one also considers the marked decrease in initiative and activeness in this group over the same period, one can make the hypothesis that these are regressive, passive patients who regard themselves in need of special consideration and care. It seems likely that at least some of the patients in Cluster I regard illness as a relief or as a means to an end (Lipowsky, 1970). Secondary gains from being ill, such as being able to expect peace and quiet, special attention and forbearance in return for presenting a whole row of health problems, seem to fit in with the picture of these patients. They certainly show a tendency to cling to the sick role (Brown & Rawlinson, 1975; Möhlen, 1979).

The patients in Cluster IV (Stable) show from the preoperative stage onwards right through until the time of the follow-up an above-average tendency to report fewer and fewer complaints. This result confirms once again how effectively their defenses work; these patients do not use their bodies as a battleground for experiencing and grappling with psychological problems, as seems to be the case with the patients in Cluster I and, though to a lesser degree, with those in Cluster III. The patients consistently managed to pay less and less attention to their hearts and the rest of their bodies from the period before the operation until the follow-up, an attitude which helps them to cope successfully with the symptoms which they certainly have, though not in a serious form.

The above-average increase in subjective physical and emotional problems in labile patients after the operation underlines the relevance of therapeutic measures, including preventive ones, to avoid setbacks during convalescence. The close interplay of financial problems, family tensions and poor psychological adjustment proves furthermore that the cooperation and assistance of social workers is urgently needed. In many surgery departments this necessity is neither recognized nor taken into account. If we want to achieve the best possible results for the patients we must provide such facilities and work together on an interdisciplinary level, for instance, using liaison psychiatry, drawing on the skills of the out-patient services and psychotherapeutic departments in rehabilitation centers, as far as these are available.

The results from this study of patients who have undergone

heart surgery also show how careful we must be to respect the psychosocial aspects in patients who are chronically ill, and how much still remains to be done for them in the future.

Reference Notes

1. Boll, A. Längerfristige psychische Anpassung Herzoperierter. Unpublished dissertation, Hamburg, 1986.
2. Lempp, F. Klinische Spätergebnisse nach Herzoperation und ihre Bedeutung für die psychosoziale Rehabilitation. Unpublished dissertation, Hamburg, 1983.

References

Adams, J. E., & Lindemann, E. Coping with long-term disability. In G. V. Coelho, D. A. Hamburg, & J. E. Adams (Eds.), *Coping and adaptation.* New York: Basic Books, 1974.
Bahnson, C. B., & Wardwell, W. I. Parent constellation and psychosexual identification in male patients with myocardial infarction. *Psychology Report Monographs Supplement,* 1962, 3-10.
Becker, R., Katz, J., Polonius, M. J., & Speidel, H. (Eds.). *Psychopathological and neurological dysfunctions following open-heart surgery.* New York: Springer, 1982.
Beckmann, D., & Richter, H. E. *Der Gießen-Test (GT).* Bern: Huber, 1972.
Brown, J. S., & Rawlinson, M. Relinquishing the sick role following open heart surgery. *Journal of Health and Social Behavior,* 1975, 16, 12-27.
Brown, J. S., & Rawlinson, M. Psychosocial status of patients randomly assigned to medical or surgical therapy for chronic stable angina. *American Journal of Cardiology,* 1979, 44, 546-554.
Cohen, R. *Systematische Tendenzen bei Persönlichkeitsbeurteilungen.* Bern: Huber, 1969.
Dahme, G., Dahme, B., Kornemann, J., Vollerts, A., & Huse-Kleinstoll, G. Fulfilment of patients expectations concerning outcome of open-heart surgery. In H. Speidel, & G.

Rodewald (Eds.), *Psychic and neurological dysfunctions after open-heart surgery.* New York: Thieme, 1980.

Dahme, B., Flemming, B., Götze, P., Huse-Kleinstoll, G., Meffert, H. J., & Speidel, H. Psycho-Somatik der Herzchirurgie. In D. Beckmann, S. Davies-Osterkamp, & J. W. Scheer (Eds.), *Medizinische Psychologie.* New York: Springer, 1982.

Davies-Osterkamp, S., Siefen, G., Möhlen, K., Müller, H., & Schlepper, M. Psychosocial situation of the open-heart surgery patient one year after operation. In B. Becker, J. Katz, M. J. Polonius, & H. Speidel (Eds.), *Psychopathological and neurological dysfunctions following open-heart surgery.* New York: Springer, 1982.

Fahrenberg, J., Selg, H., & Hampel, R. *Das Freiburger Persönlichkeitsinventar,* FPI. Göttingen: Hogrefe, 1978.

Götze, P. *Psychopathologie der Herzoperierten.* Stuttgart: Enke, 1980.

Götze, P., Flemming, B., Huse-Kleinstoll, G., Meffert, H. J., Reimer, C., & Speidel, H. Relationship between psychological syndromes before and after open-heart surgery. In R. Becker, J. Katz, J. Polonius, & H. Speidel (Eds.), *Psychopathological and neurological dysfunctions following open-heart surgery.* New York: Springer, 1982.

Götze, P., Dahme, B., & Wessel, M. Die Hamburger Schätzskala fur psychische Störungen nach Herzoperationen (HRPD). *European Archives of Psychiatry and Neurological Sciences,* 1985, *234,* 304-318.

Heller, S. S., Frank, K. A., Kornfeld, D. S., Malm, J. R., & Bowman, F. O. Psychological outcome following open-heart surgery. *Archives of Internal Medicine,* 1974, *134,* 908-914.

Heller, S. S., Frank, K. A., Kornfeld, G. S., Wilson, S. N., & Malm, J. R. Psychological and behavioral responses following coronary artery bypass surgery. In R. Becker, J. Katz, M. J. Polonius, & H. Speidel (Eds.), *Psychopathological and neurological dysfunctions following open-heart surgery.* New York: Springer, 1982.

Huse-Kleinstoll, G., Boll, A., Dahme, B., Götze, P., Meffert, H. J., Priebe, K., & Speidel, H. Die psychische Belastung kardiochirurgischer Intensivpatienten. In U. Tewes (Ed.), *Angewandte Medizinpsychologie*. Frankfurt: Klotz, 1984.

Huse-Kleinstoll, G., Boll, A., & Götze, P. Angst und Angstbewältigung vor und nach operativen Eingriffen. In P. Götze (Ed.), *Leitsymptom Angst*. New York: Springer, 1984.

Johnson, D. E. A depressive retirement syndrome. *Geriatrics*, 1958, *13*, 314-319.

Joraschky, P., & Köhle, K. Maladaption und Krankheitsmanifestation—das Streßkonzept in der psychosomatischen Medizin. In T. von Uexküll (Hrsg), *Lehrbuch der psychosomatischen Medizin* (2nd ed.). Berlin: Urban und Schwarzenberg, 1981.

von Kerekjarto, M., Meyer, A. E., & von Zerssen, D. Die HHM-Beschwerdenliste bei Patienten einer internistischen Ambulanz. *Psychosomatische Medizin Psychoanalyse*, 1972, *18*, 1-16.

Kimball, C. P. A predictive study of adjustment to cardiac surgery. *Journal of Thoracic and Cardiovascular Surgery*, 1969, *88*, 891-896.

Kimball, C. P. The experience of cardiac surgery and cardiac transplant. In J. G. Howells (Ed.), *Modern perspectives in the psychiatric aspects of surgery*. New York: Brunner & Mazel, 1976.

Lipowsky, Z. J. Physical illness, the individual and the coping process. *International Journal of Psychiatry in Medicine*, 1970, *1*, 91-102.

Lipowsky, Z. J. Physical illness and psychopathology. In Z. J. Lipowsky, D. R. Lippsitt, & P. C. Whybrow (Eds.), *Psychosomatic medicine-current-trends and clinical applications*. New York: Oxford University Press, 1977.

Lützenkirchen, N. J., Lamprecht, K., Walter, J., & Dietz, A. The sociomedical situation and personality after heart surgery. In H. Speidel, & G. Rodewald (Eds.), *Psychic and neurological dysfunctions after open-heart surgery*. Stuttgart: Thieme, 1980.

Möhlen, K. Trauer um das verlorene Herz. *Euromed 11*, 1979, *19*, 744-748.
Möhlen, K., Davies-Osterkamp, S., Müller, H., Scheld, H., & Siefen, G. Relationship between preoperative coping styles, immediate postoperative reactions and some aspects of the psychosocial situation of open-heart surgery patients one year after the operation. In R. Becker, J. Katz, M. J. Polonius, & H. Speidel (Eds.), *Psychopathological and neurological dysfunctions following open-heart surgery.* New York: Springer, 1982.
Rabiner, C. J., & Willner, A. E. Differential psychopathological and organic mental disorder at follow-up, five years after coronary bypass and cardiac valvular surgery. In H. Speidel, & G. Rodewald (Eds.), *Psychic and neurological dysfunctions after open-heart surgery.* New York: Thieme, 1980.
Reimer, C., Flemming, B., Götze, P., Huse-Kleinstoll, G., Meffert, H. J., & Speidel, H. Psychodynamic considerations and findings about patient adjustment to heart operations. In B. Becker, J. Katz, M. J. Polonius, & H. Speidel (Eds.), *Psychopathological and neurological dysfunctions following open-heart surgery.* New York: Springer, 1982.
Rodewald, G., Kalmar, P., & Krebber, H. J. Rehabilitation following open-heart surgery—from a surgeon's point of view. In B. Becker, J. Katz, M. J. Polonius, & H. Speidel (Eds.), *Psychopathological and neurological dysfunctions following open-heart surgery.* New York: Springer, 1982.
Ross, J. K., Diwell, A. E., Marsh, J., Monro, J. L., & Barker, D. J. P. Wessex cardiac surgery follow-up survey: the quality of life after operation. *Thorax,* 1978, *33,* 3-9.
Sakinofsky, I. Depression and suicide in the disabled. In D. S. Bishop (Ed.), *Behavioral problems and the disabled—assessment and management.* Baltimore: Williams & Wilkens, 1981.
Spaeth, L. *Cluster-Analyse Algorithmen.* München: Oldenbourg, 1975.
Speidel, H., Dahme, P., Flemming, B., Götze, P., Huse-Kleinstoll, G., Meffert, H. J., Rodewald, G., & Spehr, W. Psycho-

somatische Probleme in der Herzchirurgie. *Therapiewoche,* 1978, *28,* 8191-8210.

Speidel, H., & Rodewald, G. (Eds.). *Psychic and neurological dysfunctions after open-heart surgery.* New York: Thieme, 1980.

Speidel, H., Boll, A., Flemming, B., Götze, P., Huse-Kleinstoll, G., Meffert, H. J., Prüssmann, K., & Reimer, C. Problems of rehabilitation after heart surgery. In Proceedings of the 13th European Conference on Psychosomatic Research, Istanbul, 1981, 513-519.

Speidel, H. Analyse von Bedingungsfaktoren der postoperativen psychopathologischen und neurologischen Auffälligkeiten bei Herzoperierten mit extrakorporaler Zirkulation. Report to Deutsche Forschungsgemeinschaft, 1981.

Speidel, H., Boll, A., Dahme, B., & Götze, P. Psychosozialer und medizinischer Status 3-5 Jahre nach einer Herzoperation. In W. Langosch (Ed.), *Psychische Bewältigung der chronischen Herzerkrankung.* New York: Springer, 1985.

Spreen, O. Konstruktion einer Skala zur Messung der manifesten Angst in experimentellen Situationen. *Psychologische Forschung,* 1961, *26,* 105-123.

Stanton, B. A., Zyzanski, S. J., Jenkins, C. D., & Klein, M. D. Recovery after major heart surgery: medical, psychological, and work outcomes. In R. Becker, J. Katz, M. J. Polonius, & H. Speidel (Eds.), *Psychopathological and neurological dysfunctions following open-heart surgery.* New York: Springer, 1982.

Walter, P. J. (Ed.). *Return to work after coronary artery bypass surgery—psychosocial and economic aspects.* New York: Springer, 1985.

Waltz, E. M. Soziale Faktoren bei der Entstehung und Bewältigung von Krankheit—ein Überblick über die empirische Literatur. In B. Badura (Ed.), *Zum Stand sozialepidemiologischer Forschung,* edition suhrkamp. Frankfurt a. M., 1981.

2

Rescue Worker's Emotional Reactions Following a Disaster

Atle Dyregrov, Reidar Thyholdt, Jeffrey T. Mitchell

Background

This study concerns the short-term effects of stress on search and rescue personnel involved in the search, recovery and victim processes of people who were buried by an avalanche on March 5, 1986. The avalanche struck a group of 31 Norwegian army recruits and officers during a NATO exercise in northern Norway. Sixteen young men were killed, many others were wounded. Both military and civilian agencies were involved in the dangerous rescue activities which lasted several days. Helicopters transported rescue teams into the area, and personnel worked under severe weather conditions and a continuous serious threat of a new avalanche. More than 250 rescue personnel and 14 search dogs participated in rescue and recovery operations.

The civilian personnel were volunteers from various organizations, including the Red Cross. Unlike the military personnel, they were trained for search and rescue work. Survivors were extricated within a few hours; however, it took almost four days to find the last body. The frozen, dead bodies were twisted and distorted into many positions. The event constituted the greatest disaster to impact the Norwegian military forces since the Second World War. Many of the Red Cross rescuers took part in psychological debriefing sessions which were set up by local psychologists.

Introduction

Recently there has been an upsurge of interest in the effects of crisis events and stress on human service providers. Studies of police, firefighters, paramedics and other emergency personnel have brought our attention to the negative psychological consequences that ensue from the work in the border zone between life and death. Most of the research concerning rescue workers' reactions to catastrophic events has focused on manmade or technological disasters (Latane & Wheeler, 1966; Lindstrom & Lundin, 1982; Taylor & Frazer, 1982; Wilkinson, 1983; Raphael, Singh, Bradbury & Lambert, 1983; Miles, Demi & Mostyn-Aker, 1984; Weisaeth & Ersland, 1985; Jones, 1982; Durham, McCammond & Allison, 1985), although some (mostly anecdotal studies) research projects concern natural disasters (Zurcher, 1968; Laube, 1973; Ilinitch & Titus, 1977; Berah, Jones & Valent, 1984). Opinions vary on how affected rescue workers are by their work. There seems to be a consensus of opinion by the researchers that rescue workers experience short-term psychological aftereffects of the stressors they encounter in disaster work (Wilkinson, 1983; Jones, 1982; Durham et al., 1985).

Gory sights and the smell of mutilated bodies are among the many distressing factors encountered by rescue workers in a disaster. The magnitude of the event, being untrained and inadequately equipped for the work, working for long periods of time under pressure and in a state of fear for one's own life, the suffering of survivors and reactions of relatives, are all contributors to the stress emergency personnel face in the event of a disaster. Commonly noted reactions are shock and disbelief, frustration and helplessness, sadness, anger, increased anxiety and intrusive thoughts and images (recollections, images and reexperiences) which interfere with sleep. Researchers often find that rescue workers indicate changes in their lives in the aftermath of a crisis situation. Some see life as more tenuous or fragile than before (Miles et al., 1984), while others indicate a more positive change and a reevaluation of values, especially if they themselves have been in danger (Raphael et al., 1983). It has also been noted that young personnel generally experience greater stress than older workers (Taylor & Frazer, 1982; Jones, 1982).

There is considerable debate regarding the issue of long-lasting psychological after-effects. Unfortunately, there is a lack of follow-up studies. Miles et al. (1984) found no significant difference in scores on the Hopkins Symptoms Checklist (HSCL) when they compared rescue workers involved in the Hyatt Hotel disaster with normal controls. However, all five subscales and the total score were consistently higher in rescue workers. The researchers' clinical contact with rescue workers indicated that they utilized denial and repression to continue to function in their professional roles.

Jones (1982) used very broad self assessment questionnaires to measure the emotional impact of the Jonestown tragedy on those assigned the grim task of recovering the poisoned bodies. His results indicated that there was no apparent significant difference between helpers and controls 8 to 12 months following the event. Taylor and Frazer (1982) studied personnel involved in body recovery and victim identification work following the Mount Erebus aircrash in Antarctica in 1979. Their study showed that about a third of the subjects experienced some transient problems and about one-fifth maintained some symptoms after three months. The stress reactions differed according to the tasks the personnel were assigned, but persistent intrusion of particularly unpleasant sights such as disfigurements, fixed facial expressions and body contortions were reported from several workers regardless of their activity. Initially, many experienced changes in sleep, appetite, feelings, talking and social activities. Most of these changes had reverted when the workers were re-evaluated after 20 months.

On the opposing side of the issue, Lindstrom and Lundin (1982) have presented data showing more long-lasting psychological adjustment difficulties in personnel following a disastrous fire in Sweden.

This report will address the on-scene and short-term reactions of rescuers. It will also explore whether certain background factors are associated with emotional reactions.

Method

Subjects. Data in the study was collected by the first two authors at a meeting of all Red Cross personnel who were involved in rescue operations at the scene of the disaster. The meeting was held 45 days after the disaster at Vassdalen, Norway. The central Norwegian Red Cross committee had invited their personnel to this meeting to give them the opportunity to ventilate thoughts and feelings and to ask questions about the operation in Vassdalen. It was also an opportunity for the Red Cross to honor their personnel for their heroic efforts. The meeting took place six weeks after the disaster.

A questionnaire was distributed to the 100 rescuers present at the meeting. They accounted for the majority of the Red Cross personnel who worked at the Vassdalen incident. The response rate for the questionnaire was 82%. All of those present were Red Cross volunteers who had other occupations. Their Red Cross work was an avocation. There were 17 women and 65 men. Their average age was 25 years, with an age range between 17 and 55 years (SD = 6.7 years). The average length of Red Cross membership was 7 years (SD = 6 years). Thirty-five (46%) had no previous experience with rescue operations where lives had been lost, 17 (21%) had one such experience, and 29 (36%) had several.

Procedure and apparatus. A questionnaire was administered to all personnel at the end of the debriefing session, and the responders filled in the questionnaire before taking a break. The instructions from the authors were to answer the questions as openly and honestly as possible without conferring with others. They were told that the study would assist researchers in learning about the Red Cross personnel's reactions to a disastrous event.

The questionnaire was four pages long and divided into the following sections: 1) demographics including Red Cross experience; 2) role during the disaster work; 3) stress reactions during the actual rescue work; 4) post traumatic symptoms. The questionnaire was based on the author's experience with rescue workers, and on reports referred to in the introduction. The meeting was arranged on short notice, and the size of the questionnaire had to be adapted to the meeting format.

Statistics. The data from the questionnaires were coded and entered on a permanent data file. SPSS (Nie, Hull, Jenkins, Steinbrenner & Bent, 1975) was used for the statistical computations.

Results

All 82 respondents had worked at the disaster scene. The predominant functions served by the Red Cross personnel in the rescue operations were: searching in the avalanche debris (89%); digging out survivors/fatalities (30.5%); and transportation of fatalities (15.9%). Sixteen (19.5%) of the workers reported that they experienced no threat to their own lives during the operations, 46 (56.1%) experienced some threat, and 20 (24.4%) experienced a high degree of threat.

On-scene reactions. Table 1 outlines the rescuers' reports of reactions at the disaster scene.

Table 1
Experienced Reactions of Rescue Workers at the Scene

Reactions	Percentage having reaction
Fear of a new avalanche	94
Sense of helplessness	71
Thoughts about own reactions if finding somebody	71
Frustration	68
Sense of hopelessness	62
Difficulties making decisions	50
Cramp, muscle tremors	17
Nausea	8

N varies between 76 and 80.

The vast majority of the rescuers (94%) feared a new avalanche. The second most frequently reported reaction on the scene was a sense of helplessness because they were not able to do more (71%), and thoughts about how one would react if a missing person was found (71%). Frustration (68%) and a sense of hopelessness (62%) were also common reactions at the scene. Other reactions such as difficulties making decisions (50%), cramps and muscle tremors (17%) and nausea (8%) were less common. To an open question related to what they regarded as the greatest strain during the disaster, 37% spontaneously reported the danger of a new avalanche, 18% the lack of information about different aspects of the disaster organization and work, and 11% the time spent waiting before being sent into the rescue area. Many other factors were mentioned: lack of provision (food, warm shelters, etc.), physical efforts, finding and seeing bodies, etc. Personnel in a leadership role often indicated the responsibility for their personnel as the greatest strain. One of the Red Cross teams on the scene knew that a member of their own group had been overrun by the avalanche while serving his military duty. They frequently reported this knowledge to be the greatest strain during the rescue work.

Table 2 depicts the aftereffects that the rescuers had experienced in the 45 day period following the disaster.

The most common aftereffect was reexperiencing aspects of the disaster scene (75%). The majority of the rescuers (60%) also experienced greater anxiety than usual for their immediate family. They experienced images of what happened in their "mind's eye" (59%). Over one-half of the workers had difficulty in stopping themselves from talking about the event (52%), or worked hard to avoid thoughts about the event (51%). Almost half of the rescuers experienced a change in life values (47%) and a depressed mood (42%). Other more infrequent reactions are evident on Table 2.

In answer to an open-ended question about what made the greatest impression on them in connection with the disaster, the rescue workers frequently mentioned four aspects: seeing the dead soldiers, the loss of young people, the magnitude of the event and the power of nature's forces, and the memorial service arranged by the military when all the missing soldiers had been found. Some rescuers also commented on the good teamwork within the Red Cross teams.

Table 2
Post-Event Reactions of Rescue Workers

Reactions	Percentage having reaction
Reexperiencing the event	75
Anxiety for one's closest family	60
Mental images of the event ("flashbacks")	59
Extremely strong need to talk about event	52
Avoiding thoughts about the event	51
Change of life values	47
Depressed mood (sadness)	42
General anxiety	39
Resentment about lack of acknowledgment of rescue efforts	35
Lack of understanding from family	31
Difficulties concentrating	27
Lack of energy	23
Sleep disturbances	23
Difficulties returning to usual line of work	17
Avoiding contacts with others	6
Nightmares	4

N varies between 77 and 80.

Rescuer reactions at the scene and in the 45 day period following the rescue operations were not related to age or to years of membership in the Red Cross in any clearly identifiable manner.

On scene reactions did not significantly differ between the two sexes, although the women's mean values generally were higher than the men. However, the two sexes differed on most post traumatic reactions. Women reported significantly more depressed moods ($F = 18.46$, $df = 1/77$, $p < .001$), nightmares ($F = 12.84$, $df = 1/75$, $p < .005$), anxiety for loved ones ($F = 8.98$, $df = 1/77$, $p < .01$), sleep disturbances ($F = 8.32$, $df = 1/77$, $p < .01$), isolation from others ($F = 7.94$, $df = 1/76$, $p < .05$), difficulties concentrating ($F = 6.08$, $df = 1/77$, $p < .05$), mental images of the event ($F = 5.63$, $df = 1/78$, $p < .05$), lack of energy ($F = 5.60$, $df = 1/76$, $p < .05$), anxiety for other things ($F = 4.87$, $df = 1/75$, $p < .05$), and difficulties returning to their usual work ($F = 4.01$, $df = 1/77$, $p < .05$) than the men.

Those who were in close contact with one or more dead soldiers retrospectively indicated significantly more thoughts about how they would react if they found somebody ($F = 7.04$, $df = 1/78$, $p < .01$). They also experienced significantly more difficulties concentrating ($F = 4.41$, $df = 1/77$, $p < .05$) in the period following the disaster. Those who indicated that they experienced a serious threat to their life indicated more anxiety for their loved ones ($F = 5.77$, $df = 2/78$, $p < .01$), more general anxiety ($F = 3.25$, $df = 2/76$, $p < .05$), more irritability ($F = 3.18$, $df = 2/77$, $p < .05$). Those rescuers involved in the search for the missing ($N = 71$) experienced significantly more intrusive images than those ($N = 9$) rescuers not involved in this task ($F = 4.21$, $df = 1/79$, $p < .05$).

When comparing reactions between rescuers with a leadership role ($N = 16$) during the operations (team leader, line search leader, etc.) with those without leadership responsibility ($N = 63$), the only significant difference was found to be the reaction regarding "lack of acknowledgment for work done." Leaders indicated significantly greater lack of acknowledgment than non-leaders ($F = 4.23$, $df = 1/78$, $p < .05$).

Discussion

Rescuers experienced symptoms of fear and distress at the disaster scene. Fear of a new avalanche was the most commonly reported reaction, but feelings of helplessness, frustration and hopelessness were also common, as were thoughts about their own reactions if they found a person in the snow. Their answer to an open-ended question on what they regarded as the greatest strain during the disaster work also pointed to the fear of a new avalanche, as well as the lack of information regarding different aspects of the situation. In the period following the disaster, intrusive symptoms were the most common reactions (reexperiencing the event, images of the event), along with anxiety for one's close family. About half of the respondents acknowledged avoiding thoughts about the event. In answer to an open question about what made the greatest impression on them in the disaster, rescuers answered: seeing the dead people, the loss of young people, the magnitude of the event, and the memorial event which followed later. When analyzing how demographic and background data were related to on-scene reactions and aftereffects, the most conspicuous findings were that the women reported significantly more symptoms following the disaster than men.

In most disaster situations, rescuers are not usually faced with such an imminent danger of death as they experienced in Vassdalen. Almost 100% experienced fear of a new avalanche. This fear was increased by an inadequate method accounting for personnel entering or leaving the search area. One rescuer said on this matter, "I would not have been found until spring came." Rescue personnel were also distressed by a lack of work light and avalanche guards, and the lack of adequate information in the probability of a new avalanche. Although faced with this fear, the personnel were able to carry out their duties in an impressive manner. Some of the rescuers at the meeting indicated that they made active cognitive attempts to cope with the fear: "If everything has gone well for two days, it will go well for an additional day."

The rescuers were faced with assisting the injured and recovering the bodies (frequently mutilated) of the dead who were healthy, vibrant people just a few seconds before the avalanche struck. The sense of death and destruction evidently caused similar feelings of helplessness, hopelessness and frustration as found by researchers in other studies of disaster workers (Raphael et al., 1983; Miles et al., 1984).

The degree of frustration experienced at the scene also resulted from a lack of supplies and warm rest facilities, poor interagency cooperation, conflicting orders from command staff and a chaotic situation at the scene, especially in the early stages of the operation.

The personnel commented, both in the questionnaire and

at the meeting, that what they had experienced first hit them when they came home, and the operation was over. Their reactions are consistent with those found in other studies (Wilkinson, 1983; Durham et al., 1985) when recollections of the event have been found the most common symptom. Seeing and handling dead bodies, often close to one's own age, is a very powerful event, and it may trigger mental images and anxiety in the rescuers. However, when those who indicated that they had close contact with the dead were compared to those with less contact with the dead, significant differences were not found in the frequency to which they had experienced intrusive mental images. There was, however, a slightly higher mean score for reexperiencing the event as well as for most of the other symptoms in those with close contact with the dead (cfr. 8). The only difference between these two groups that reached statistical significance was difficulty concentrating. The close contact group reported more problems concentrating than those who had limited contact with the dead ($F = 4.41$, $df = 1/77$, $p < .05$). Our clinical experience from working with rescuers and others who have witnessed a critical incident situation often has shown that difficulty concentrating originates from intrusive material entering the brain's information processing faculties often without conscious awareness. It is evident from these results that being a bystander and a witness to body recovery is sufficient to trigger reexperiences and intrusive images from the event. One did not have to touch the corpses personally to be affected. The bodies were often twisted in highly unnatural positions, thus creating grotesque sights which were later replayed in the minds of the rescuers. Besides the sights of the recovered bodies, the situation at large seemed to have made a deep and lasting impression on the rescuers. The magnitude of the disaster and the meaningless death of so many young men helped to engrave the event in their memories.

On the basis of the authors' clinincal experience with other populations experiencing critical incidents in their lives, a question about anxiety for one's loved ones was included in the questionnaire. Few studies before have addressed this aspect.

The results in this study indicated that 60% of the rescuers reported that they had experienced this reaction to some degree. One of the men described his reactions in the following way: "For a while following the disaster I often had to enter my daughter's bedroom to check if she was OK and if she slept. This happened many times during a night. While riding in my car my daughter once fell asleep. When I saw her sitting there quite limp and lifeless, I was back at the disaster scene again."

Both the anxiety for loved ones and the general anxiety following the Vassdalen disaster depict a loss of invulnerability in rescuers which parallels that of victims and victims' families in the aftermath of a range of traumatic events (Dyregrov & Matthiesen, 1987a). Most people live in an illusion of invulnerability ("it won't happen to me") that is partially and at times totally shattered when one is exposed to traumatic situations or the forces of nature. The results in this study also showed that those who indicated that they experienced a serious threat to their lives felt more general anxiety and fear for their loved ones and a greater sense of vulnerability. Some of the respondents commented on how helpless one is when nature's forces strike; that people the same age as themselves died, and that they might have lost their lives if a new avalanche had occurred. The rescuers obviously experienced some degree of identification with the dead and their families. Faced with such large scale death and powerful natural forces, people experience helplessness and what Lifton (1967) has termed the "death imprint," which consists of memories and images of the disaster associated with death, dying and destruction.

The increased anxiety or vulnerability was paralleled by a reported change in life values by nearly half of the rescuers. The study does not give us detail on what kind of changes took place. The relatively sparse qualitative material indicates that materialistic values were de-emphasized, while non-materialistic values, such as "closeness to others," importance of friends and family, etc., were upgraded. The intensity of emotions following such an event seems to increase both the reporting of symptoms and more "positive" emotions that emphasize the value of human life and bonding between people. The results of the current study confirm the observations and findings of others (Wilkinson, 1983; Raphael et al., 1983; Miles et al., 1984; Jones, 1982). The value of being able to help others seems to be reflected both in the questionnaire answers and comments made by the respondents. The feelings of helplessness, hopelessness and frustration felt on the scene suggest a high value placed by rescuer personnel on doing something to help others. The fact that many rescuers mentioned the waiting time before being either flown into the area or before being put into active work as the greatest strain, also indicates the strong need of being able to help others, and the frustration felt when unable to fulfill this need. From other research it is well known that helplessness over not being able to help is often experienced as highly stressful by rescuers (Raphael et al., 1983).

The lack of acknowledgment felt by many (especially leaders) added to the feelings of frustration. One of the leaders said he felt disillusioned and had lost some of his motivation for Red Cross work because of the lack of acknowledgment he felt he and his personnel experienced both on the scene and afterwards.

A surprising result was the lack of association between amount of experience and age, and emotional symptoms. This may reflect the highly unusual magnitude of the event, where age and experience were insufficient to deal with the situation. It is also possible that those with more experience were more exposed to trauma than those with less experience. Another explanation might be that the younger and more inexperienced workers have been more able to deal with the event in debriefing sessions and better able to utilize peer support than the others.

Earlier research reports have been sparse concerning sex differences in rescuers' reactions. The results in this study show a clear difference in reported post-disaster reactions among the two sexes. From other research it is well known that women generally report more emotional reactions than men following critical events (Dyregrov & Matthiesen, 1987b). It is interesting to note that rescuers show the same pattern.

Further research is necessary to learn more about the possible explanations for this distinct difference (whether it is caused by denial or conscious under-reporting of reactions by men due to differences in sociocultural socialization or upbringing, a different set of coping mechanisms in men and women, etc.). Further research in this area might disclose what practical implications the differences have for training and follow-up debriefing work.

Group cohesion and group support seemed important in supporting and motivating the rescuers in this stress situation. Both in the questionnaire and during the meeting of all the personnel, the value of the group in sustaining the efforts at the scene and in supporting each other in the post-disaster period was emphasized. Rescue workers often have a need to talk of what has happened (Lindstrom & Lundin, 1983), and may even experience difficulties ceasing their discussions about the event (see Table 2). In general this study supports the previously researched conclusion that rescue personnel perceive talking as most helpful in dealing with distressing thoughts and feeling (Miles et al., 1984).

The study format and number of respondents require caution regarding the conclusions to be drawn from this study. However, the results warrant further research in various areas to understand how tragic events influence the well-being of voluntary and career helpers.

Conclusion

Disaster creates emotional upheaval in most rescuers. Ordinary people experience normal psychological reactions in response to an abnormal event. Psychological debriefing sessions (Mitchell, 1983) are strongly recommended as a routine in rescue organizations following critical incidents. Debriefings provide rescuers with a method for alleviating immediate stress responses and preventing long-term difficulties in coping with the event. Further research is needed to understand the natural healing process which takes place within the normal support system of the rescuers, as well as the process within more formalized methods of helping (psychological debriefing). Care must also be taken to give the voluntary personnel acknowledgment for the great amount of energy and effort they put into the rescue work. Dedicated efforts are needed within voluntary and career organizations to assure adequate personnel care and assistance in the event of disaster.

References

Berah, E. F., Jones, H. J., & Valent, P. The experience of a mental health team involved in the early phase of a disaster. *Australia-New Zealand Journal of Psychiatry,* 1984, *18,* 354-358.

Durham, T. W., McCammond, S. L., & Allison, E. J. The psychological impact of disaster on rescue personnel. *Annual of Emergency Medicine,* 1985, *14,* 664-668.

Dyregrov, A., & Matthiesen, S. B. Anxiety and vulnerability in parents following the death of an infant. *Scandinavian Journal of Psychology,* 1987, *28,* 16-25.

Dyregrov, A., & Matthiesen, S. B. Similarities and differences in mothers' and fathers' grief following the death of an infant. *Scandinavian Journal of Psychology,* 1987, *28,* 1-5.

Ilinitch, R. C., & Titus, M. P. Caretakers as victims: the big Thompson flood, 1976. Abstracts of master's thesis. Smith College Study of Social Work, 1977, *48,* 67-68.

Jones, D. R. Secondary disaster victims: the emotional effects of recovering and identifying human remains. *American Journal of Psychiatry,* 1982, *142,* 4-12.

Latane, B., & Wheeler, L. Emotionality and reactions to disaster. *Journal of Experimental Social Psychology,* 1966, Suppl. 1, 95-102.

Laube, J. Psychological reactions of nurses in disaster. *Nursing Research,* 1973, *22,* 343-347.

Lifton, R. J. *Death in life.* New York: Basic Books, 1967.

Lindstrom, B., & Lundin, T. Yrkesmassig eksponering for katastrof. *Nord Psykiatrisk Tidsskr,* 1982, Suppl. 6, 1-44.

Miles, M. S., Demi, A. S., & Mostyn-Aker, P. Rescue workers' reactions following the Hyatt hotel disaster. *Death Education,* 1984, *8,* 315-331.

Mitchell, J. When disaster strikes... the critical incident stress debriefing process. *Journal of Emergency Medicine Services*, 1983, Winter, 36-39.

Nie, N. H., Hull, C. H., Jenkins, J. G., Steinbrenner, K., & Bent, D. H. *SPSS. Statistical package for the social sciences*. New York: McGraw Hill, 1975.

Raphael, B., Singh B., Bradbury, L., & Lambert, F. Who helps the helpers? The effects of a disaster on the rescue workers. *Omega*, 1983, *14*, 9-20.

Taylor, A. W., & Frazer, A. G. The stress of post-disaster body handling and victim identification work. *Journal of Human Stress*, 1982, *8*, 4-12.

Weisaeth, L., & Ersland, S. Redningspersonell: stressreaksjoner under innsats og psykiske følger. I Retterstøl, N. & Weisaeth, L. Katastrofer og kriser. Oslo: Universitetsforlaget, 1985.

Wilkinson, C. B. Aftermath of a disaster: the collapse of the Hyatt Regency Hotel skywalks. *American Journal of Psychiatry*, 1983, *140*, 1135-1139.

Zurcher, L. A. Social-psychological functions of ephemeral roles: a disaster work crew. *Human Organization*, 1968, *27*, 281-297.

3

The Sick Person in a Field of Tension in Modern Society— Psychosis and Carcinoma as a Counterpart

Wolfgang Jacob

In this paper I shall try to give a survey about the "irrationality of carcinoma" as part of a process of "Organ-Psychosis" (Meng, 1944), and compare it with the phenomena of schizophrenia.

Gaetano Benedetti (1975), in his paper "Curative Factors in Psychotherapy with Schizophrenic Patients" pointed out the following:

1. "The dynamics of the therapist's unconscious, as shown by some of his dreams."
2. "The therapeutic fantasy."
3. "The 'mirror phenomenon' in the psychotherapy of schizophrenia."
4. "The integration of love and aggression in the patient and in the therapist."

If we try to understand schizophrenia and carcinoma as phenomena striving in opposite directions, then first of all it is possible to show the opposing movement of the therapeutic experience with reference to Benedetti's statements:

Point 1) I do not know, at least from the initial phase of the psychotherapeutic accompaniment of a cancer patient, of any manifest dream thematic material on the part of the therapist, which can be directly related to the unconscious of the patient.

Point 2) In the case of cancer patients this point deals with the therapeutic fantasy not of the psychiatrist but of the oncologist. However, here we do know of the normal case of the exceptionally aggressive behavior which the doctor who has not been schooled in psychoanalysis exhibits towards the cancer patient in particular, a behavior which comes from the unconscious and which must be called "anti-therapeutic." Of course, this situation is influenced, among other things, by the aggressive organic character of the disease.

Point 3) If we try to recognize the equivalent of a mirror function of the therapist in the carcinoma therapy, something completely different from the experience gained with schizophrenia becomes apparent (I will return to this point later on).

Point 4) The transference dynamics of an integration of love and aggression in the patient and in the doctor are expressed more here and now; that is to say, they appear in the beginning more in factual and spatial shifts and changes, which occupy the doctor and the patient, than in a spiritual or dream world.

In this paper, I would like first to consider my further comments on these points from the aspect of *hypertrophic* realism (Jacob, 1985), which governs the scene of the disease of cancer in contrast to that of delusions, and which habitually fills the cancer patient in his conception of the world and in his being and which becomes evident not only in the somatic therapy but also in the therapeutic accompaniment. The irrationality of this hypertrophic realism in the world of the patient, in contrast to the irrationality in the fantasy and dream world of the schizophrenic, deserves special attention in this context. A reality becomes pathogenic for the patient, which Viktor von Weizsäcker has called "delusion of material" (1957).

Second, I would like to try to consider the irrational phenomena which we come across in Benedetti's four principle points. An additional step will be to look at the therapeutic consequences in light of Benedetti's points. The dream activity of the therapist, that is, the involvement of his unconscious in the therapy, is not only necessary in order to check his countertransference but, as Benedetti can show, precisely a therapeutic factor in the treatment of the schizophrenic.

Benedetti's second point has to do with therapeutic fantasy. Without it I feel that no therapeutic success is at all possible. Quite generally speaking it is an element of the art of medicine, even if, as is the case in purely somatic treatment, it is forced into the Procrustean bed of strict scientific proof. A poor doctor is not only one who does not have mastery of the method, but also one who incorrectly applies the only method which seems right to him. Incorrectly here means: applying it according to a narrowly defined rule instead of in accordance with confident knowledge and selection of what is best and most useful for the patient here and now. He knows nothing of the "illness will" (Groddeck, 1983) or the "death" instinct (Freud, 1976) of the patient.

This is where true medical experience, gained from the differences among people and diseases, differs from merely performing a skill according to a set of rules. This difference manifests itself at the latest in the perplexity of the therapy, which finally fails completely in the advanced stages of the disease. But here again we encounter the irrationality of the disease process, the irrationality of a "psychosis" in the diseased organ, concretely: the irrational productivity of the carcinoma. According to scientific rules, the only remaining possibility in later stages is to allow the disease's raging destructive process, which can no longer be rationally "controlled," to run its course in a kind of therapeutic powerlessness and to palliatively relieve symptoms of the disease such as pain.

Thus ends the life fate, the fate figure of the cancer patient as a "disease to death," the death of the whole organism, which in turn is diametrically opposed to the death fate of the soul of the schizophrenic. He experiences his death fate, his "half plunge into death" (Weizsäcker, 1949) and ends up in a total crisis. The cancer patient, on the other hand, resigns himself to his rationally unalterable fate without the conflict, which has been taken over by the organ, appearing directly in the form of the "psychosis." The incomprehensible which comes to light in the disease phenomena of schizophrenia stands opposite to the incomprehensible of the malignant tumor growth in the cancer patient, whereas the life and experience realm of the cancer patient seems to be overly well-adjusted and overly rational. It is precisely this state of disease that I call *"hypertrophic realism."*

Whereas the dream and fantasy world of the person suffering from delusions, even if it expresses itself monomaniacally in the disease, has no limits in its creativity. In comparison, in the case of the cancer patient, except for the account of a sociobiography which is usually perceived as having been extremely painful and depressive, there is virtually nothing which our rationally oriented everyday life could not offer us. The therapist who is inexperienced in dealing with the seriously organically ill, especially with cancer patients, allows himself to be deceived by this hypertrophic realism. He refers to the emptiness of the emotional realm of expression which he encounters in contrast to neurosis, as "alexithymia." In other words, the carcinoma patient, just like the schizophrenic, reacts refractorily to classic psychoanalytical neurosis therapy.

Thus in wide circles of psychotherapy, schizophrenia as well as carcinoma are still felt to be largely unsuitable for any psychotherapeutic intervention at all. The understanding of psychodynamics, which was developed from the neurosis model, is able to do justice neither to the main emphasis of the psychodynamic disease process in the case of schizophrenia nor to the disease of cancer. In both cases the therapist capitulates in the face of the incomprehensible. This is also and particularly true of the irrational, which is hidden behind the phenomenon of the "hypertrophic realism" or the "alexithymia" (Rad, 1985) of the cancer patient!

Before I attempt to have a look at the social dimension of the opposition in the form of appearance of schizophrenia as opposed to cancer, I would like to point out a phenomenon stressed by Benedetti (1975): The schizophrenic can only perceive the contact with the therapist in a depersonalized and projected way. The therapist has to actually keep himself from being entangled in the multi-faceted net of messages and communication fantasy of his schizophrenic patient. But for the schizophrenic, the experience presents itself in the opposite way: "I am an amoeba to which everyone can enter." The patient feels trapped by others. The boundaries of his ego are open on all sides, "everyone can enter"!

The cancer patient, like the schizophrenic, is also unable to demarcate himself, especially from the people around him. However, for all outward appearances, even right before the disaster strikes, he seems like an intact, completely adjusted, realistic, rationally thinking human being who has long since discarded virtually all realms of his fantasy. In fact, even any sentiment of religious fantasy which goes beyond the rational experience of a rationally founded moral virtue is discarded. Nothing seems to be able to withstand this discursive and at the same time destructive rational thinking, except for the altruistic belief. This altruistic belief is lived vicariously for others, in the morality of a truly rational enlightenment and arrangement of all realms of life. This phenomenological world of the cancer patient is not only mirrored in the "alexithymia experience" of the therapist, but it even mirrors the hypertrophic rationalism of a world view, which largely determines our everyday life in society.

In reality the irrationality of one's own life concept, with the tacit approval of the patient himself, was condemned to powerlessness and buried early on. The cancer patient, as L. LeShan says, has long since been unable "to sing his own song" (1977). His altruism, which is diametrically opposed to the phenomenologically apparent absolute egocentrism of the schizophrenic, corresponds to an ideal ego which is sustained by high moral and rationalized values, which is fully entangled in the world of rational realism and which has totally dissociated or even alienated itself from its fantasy-minded and dreaming (we would say irrational-minded) self, which has long since been buried and condemned to powerlessness.

But what, in contrast to the treatment of schizophrenia, is the therapeutic mirror for the personality of the cancer patient? How can therapeutically effective communication be achieved here, comparable to the conditions of the therapeutic communication which is able to have a healing effect on the schizophrenic's illness fate, which had seemed inaccesible before?

There are several important and essential differences here between the two diseases, whose polar structure is perhaps of help to us with our question:

1. Cancer is a disease which manifests itself organically; psychosis exhibits a few changes in brain metabolism which can be influenced by drugs, but there is no life-threatening destruction process of the organ.
2. Where delusions, i.e., realms of thoughts which strike other people as incomprehensible, can emerge, malignant growth is more likely to subside. (Statistics have shown that the schizophrenic is less susceptible to oncological diseases [Booth, Note 1].)
3. It is not the socially destructive irrationality as seen in the person suffering from delusions, which is the basis of his ego-fragmentation, that disturbs and burdens the therapeutic possibilities of communication with the cancer patient. Rather, it is the fact that the alter ego is rationally overly adjusted and the actual self, which upon closer examination is usually completely weak and isolated, and cannot escape from the rut of everyday life. This realm is also shaped by a hypertrophically, rationalistically oriented general life realm in our society; whereas, the so-called healthy members of this life realm disregard the constraints of such a world (which has been rationalized down to the last detail), by reacting contradictorily. That is, they react anti-

logically or with the forces of the pervasive "mendacity of life" (Weizsäcker, 1957). By breaking out of this realm, the cancer patient takes this pathologically degenerate realm completely seriously, and he has long since incorporated it into his ideal ego and his moral value system. The biography of the cancer patient Sigmund Freud is an eloquent example of this disease development (Jacob, 1985).

For all these reasons schizophrenia and cancer still seem to the inexperienced psychotherapist as being as inaccessible as neuroses seem to the general practitioner. Both diseases look like erratic blocks in the otherwise rather optimistic therapeutic scene of neuroses, pseudo-neuroses or of the so-called classic psychosomatic diseases. There is very little evidence that this will change in the near future.

Nevertheless, a certain change in the therapeutic interest and in the focus of therapeutic work is becoming apparent, not only in the advances in recognizing biochemical and immunobiological connections involved in these two diseases, but this change also shows up in the fact that we are turning to and exposing ourselves to what had previously seemed incomprehensible in the encounter with patients, that is, in the therapeutic communication with the patient in a manner not assumed by an objectification and psychopathological understanding. An example of this from the pain situation: Here hypertrophic realism of medicine as a science is reflected at the same time in the interpretation of the illness phenomenon. The real pain sensation and the infinite oversensitiveness of the schizophrenic used to be completely denied by traditional psychiatrists and certainly not heeded. How could the delusions of painful sensations actually be painful for the patient in reality? The hypersensitive pain sensations of the hypochondriac were denied all credibility.

Today many aspects of the previously incomprehensible phenomena have become accessible through a better psychodynamic understanding of the biographical connection. The frequently unbearable pain suffered by the cancer patient can as a rule be explained rationally by the organic findings and can be palliatively relieved by means of pain medication. And yet, looking at the phenomenon that a cancer patient whose lumbar vertebral column is literally permeated with metastases and for whom drugs "do not help any more," how can we explain that in such a case a simple hypnotic suggestion not only relieves his unbearable pain for days but at the same time it also greatly improves his responsiveness to pain-relieving drugs? In the hypnotic stage this patient had fulfilled a longstanding wish to stretch out luxuriously on the beach and to look up at the blue sky (Bahnson, Note 2).

We encounter a phenomenon here that has not yet been sufficiently considered for organic disease. The phenomenon involves the ordering power of symbolic notions and wishes, which do not fit into the general, strictly rationally oriented world of the allegedly healthy and capable member of an average society. These notions include wishes that appear like a "mental disarray and contradictoriness" and anti-logic (Weizsäcker, 1957). The patient had not dared to acknowledge and allow these irrational basics of his healthy life.

Now the *symbolic character* of these two diseases should be studied in the psychodynamic realm; but that should be a further step to which I can only refer here. Instead allow me to return once again to Benedetti's third point, the mirror function of the therapist. For the cancer patient the points of contact with the social institution seem to play an exceptional role. The attempt to psychotherapeutically accompany the cancer patient meets with unexpected resistance even and especially where the somatic treatment has reached its limits and oncological treatment tells us that further somatic treatment seems to be neither indicated nor reasonable.

The therapist here appears as a pathogenic mirror of the futility and hopelessness of the disease process, and not only because he himself fears the disease he is treating. In this fear his unconscious so strongly reflects back onto the patient the negative social fears and destructions associated with cancer, which should be avoided through the basis of the treatment, that any positive therapeutic mirror function is subjected to a social verdict.

Nowhere is the purism of a rational therapy control, even where it must be seen as futile, carried out so radically as in oncological therapy. Classic psychoanalysis also follows similar principles of control here, as the analyses of the cancer patient F. Zorn can show us (1977).

A gap was made in the wall of this social resistance (Weizsäcker, 1949) which conceals the real mirror function of the therapy, for the first time in the fifties, through the efforts of an American psychotherapist group under Gotthard Booth. Booth and other authors have been able to show that the social resistance, which Viktor von Weizsäcker felt to be invincible, does not seem to be completely invincible in individual cases. But at what price?

Here, too, one cannot avoid turning one's attention to the social perspective, as it was probably first included by M. Siirala in schizophrenia of the individual in its relationship to schizophrenia of the general public: This particular relation must also be sought in conjunction with cancer. Gotthard Booth (1979) presented it in his posthumously published work "Cancer Epidemic—The Shadow of the Conquest of Nature." Here we cannot go into a presentation of the social pathological process of cancer and its social irrationalisms. It seems that the organ psychosis of the carcinoma turns out to be an equivalent of social pathologically-working dynamics.

Reference Note

1. Booth, G. Personality and disease in cancer, lecture, 1965.
2. Bahnson, C.B. Personal Communication, 1972.

References

Benedetti, G. Curative factors in psychotherapy with schizophrenic patients. In *Schizophrenia 75 - proceedings of the Vth international symposium on the psychotherapy of schizophrenia.* Oslo: Universitetsforlaget, 1975, 15-27.

Booth, G. *The cancer epidemic: shadow of the conquest of nature.* New York: Edwin Mellen Press, 1979.

Freud, S. *Jenseits des Lustprinzips.* GW Bd. XIV, 6. Aufl. Frankfurt: Fischer, 1976.

Groddeck, G. *Krankheit als Symbol* (Hrsg.: Siefert, H.). Frankfurt: Fischer, 1983.

Jacob, W. Aufklärung, psychische Führung. In *Handbuch für innere medizin,* Bd. IV/4. Heidelberg: Springer, 1985.

Jacob, W. Kultur und Psychoanalyse. In *Daseinsanalyse.* Basel: Karger, 1985, 2, 37-50.

LeShan, L. *You can fight for your life.* New York: M. Evans & Co., 1977.

Meng, H. *Psyche und Hormon.* Bern: Huber, 1944.

Rad, M. v. *Alexithymie.* Springer, 1985.

Weizsäcker, V. v. *Pathosophie.* Göttinger: Vandenhoeck & Ruprecht, 1957.

Weizsäcker, V. v. *Begegnungen und Entscheidungen.* Stuttgart: K. F. Köhler, 1949.

Weizsäcker, V. v. Der Widerstand bei der Behandlung von Organkranken mit ßemerkungen über Werke von Jean-Paul Sartre. *In Psyche. Zeitschr./Tiefenpsych.* Marz: Heft, 1949, II., Jg. 4., 481-498.

Zorn, F. *"Mars."* Munchen: Kindler, 1977.

4

Considerations for the Impact of Medical Therapy on Quality of Life

Margit von Kerekjarto

Doubts about the effectiveness of many medical interventions are not new. The essential argument advanced by critics is that patients' health is influenced only to a minor extent by the technologically based medical care they receive. My intention is to try to evaluate the impact of modern medical technology on quality of life (QOL), with and without adjuvant psychosocial intervention.

Currently I am working with an oncology department. With three of my co-workers, we are providing a type of consultation-liaison service for ward patients as well as out-patients. We provide psycho-social care for severely ill and dying patients as well as crisis-intervention, if necessary, after patients first hear of a diagnosis of breast cancer, Hodgkin's disease or some other malignant-related illness in oncology. Thus we are confronted daily with the conflict between necessary medical technical treatment and the impact that treatment has on patients.

First of all, we must determine how the QOL concept may best be conceptualized. Gerson (1976) defines quality of life: "QOL is measured by the degree to which an individual succeeds in accomplishing his desires despite the constraints put upon him by a hostile or indifferent nature, God or social order" (p. 794). Another definition from Burt and co-workers (1978) is:

An individual's evaluation of his/her QOL derives from the level of consumption of socially valued goods and services relative to social norms....the extent to which an individual feels he has the power to determine his individual well-being within society. (p. 367)

In the last half decade there has been a rapid growth in the literature concerned with measuring QOL. Two major studies (Campbell, Converse & Rogers, 1976; Andrews & Withey, 1976) provided the basis for the current state of research into social indicators of QOL. Both extended existing models of QOL to include, in addition to measures of general satisfaction and positive and negative affect, measures of satisfaction with specific domains of activity. These domains cover aspects of an individual's life, such as health, marriage, job environment, and material circumstances. The implicit assumption is that these are valid indicators of QOL.

Today we know at least four principal weaknesses of objective indicators, which have restricted their utility:

1. vagueness in determining the basic dimensions of what constitutes a high or low QOL;
2. disagreements about which indicators are relevant;
3. little or no concern about ability to relate inputs to outcomes;
4. no understanding of the association between the objective conditions of life and the subjective perception of these conditions.

Subjective social indicators of QOL used in studies produced more consistent findings than those that used objective social indicators. Subjective indicators of the QOL have included terms like "happiness," overall satisfaction with life or global well-being. These positive feelings appear fairly stable over time and correlate moderately well with each other.

Many studies have shown that positive descriptions of one's marriage and family situation are good, if not the best, predictors of overall happiness and satisfaction with life.

In general, the major determinants of high subjective QOL appear to be positive, close and stable social relationships. In addition, the smaller the gap between expectation and objective circumstances, the greater the level of subjectively reported QOL.

The only exception involves the impact of health on QOL. Good or poor health is not, in general, closely related to happiness or satisfaction with life. Campbell et al. (1976) found that almost one-half of those people who report disabilities severe enough to prevent them from doing "a lot of things" are unwilling to say that they are dissatisfied in any degree with their health, and a small number of them (6%) insist that they are completely satisfied with it.

Health variables explain between 4-16% of the variance in the QOL of older people.

In the following, let us focus on criteria for evaluating the impact of medical technologies on the QOL.

I did a MEDLARS search using QOL as keyword and checked the literature from 1976 onwards using the *Index Medicus* and *Psychological Abstracts*. For my selection of relevant articles, I screened about 60-70 listings, concentrating on original studies and leaving out review-articles. I found approximately 20 articles dealing directly with issues of QOL. A few weeks earlier, Najman and Levine (1981) offered a nearly identical selection (see Tables 1 to 3).

Table 1 shows the questions investigated by the different studies. The summarized results of these studies were so negative in spite of impressive medical technology that substantial changes in health care would be necessary in order to improve QOL.

Table 1
Questions Addressed by Studies Which Use Quality of Life Criteria to Justify the Delivery of Health Care.

What factors over time predict changes in the QOL of burn victims?
What drug regimen for breast cancer minimizes side effects?
Is employment status an adequate QOL indicator for coronary artery bypass surgery (C.A.B.S.)?
How does chemotherapy for breast cancer affect the QOL?
What is the QOL of persons surviving a liver transplant?
Do dialysis patients have a worse QOL than those with kidney transplants?
Does exstrophy closure improve the QOL of patients?
Does an endurance conditioning program increase the QOL?
What is the QOL of children and adolescents with a kidney transplant?
Does open-heart (largely valve replacement) surgery improve the QOL?
What is the QOL of survivors of a total gastrectomy?
What is the QOL of newborn children surviving surgery for intestinal obstruction?
What is the improvement in the QOL of older persons receiving a total hip replacement?
Does C.A.B.S. improve the QOL?
Does intestinal bypass surgery for the morbidly obese improve their QOL?
Does radiation for bone metastases improve the QOL?
Does microvascular bypass surgery improve the QOL?
What is the QOL of infants vigorously resuscitated for perinatalasphyxia?
What is the effect of knowledge of a terminal diagnosis on the QOL?
Do different chemotherapeutic regimens for advanced breast cancer have different QOL effects?
Does colostomy irrigation improve the QOL?
Does less aggressive chemotherapy for myeloid leukemia improve the QOL?
Does an internal ileal reservoir improve the QOL of ileostomy patients?

In Table 2 the criteria used to assess the improvement of QOL are listed. As you can see, most of the studies used only objective indicators, and are thus of doubtful validity. Only Blades (1979), Meyerowitz (1980), and Campbell et al. (1976) were exceptions.

Table 2
Evaluating the Impact of Medical Care and Technologies on the Quality of Life (QOL)

QOL criteria used in different studies	Obj[1]	Obj[3] Subj[2] and Subj.
Hours worked, income, job status, joint function, psychosocial adaptation and self-perception	x	x
Side effects like nausea, vomiting, depression	x	
Work status, desire to work, perceived limits	x	
Patient judges changes in marriage/family/sex/activity level, etc.		x
Clinical judges return to normal activity, percent time hospitalized	x	
Employment status, activity level, sexual function, depression, brain dysfunction and physical symptoms	x	
Sexual activity, having children, working, emotional difficulties	x	
Requirement of food, clothing, shelter, health, interpersonal relationships	x	
Whether school or job, number of social relationships, depression, fear of kidney rejection	x	
Shortness of breath, limitations to normal activity, employment status, sexual relationships	x	
Nutrition, oesophagitis, other disabling symptoms	x	

Considerations for the Impact of Medical Therapy

QOL criteria used in different studies	Obj[1]	Obj[3] Subj[2] and Subj.
Height, weight, malabsorption, I.Q., visual/motor perception	x	
Range of movement, pain, mobility, Adjective Checklist (A.D.L.)	x	
Work status and number of hours worked	x	
Temper, working capacity, leisure time activity, interpersonal relationships, sexual activity	x	
Pain relief and clinician's judgment of ability to care for self	x	
Relief from symptoms, improved functioning, reduced dementia, clinician's subjective judgment	x	
Neurologic abnormality, psycholinguistic ability and normal development	x	
Clinical judgment about control of symptoms, interpersonal relationships and manner of death	x	
Level of activity, pain, nausea, appetite, anxiety, perceived benefits of treatment, feelings of well-being, mood	x	x
Accidental bowel actions, wind, restriction of diet and social activities, normal "life"	x	
Judgment about symptom and morbidity control, normal "life"	x	
Judgments about the ability to live normally	x	

[1] Objective social indicator used
[2] Subjective social indicators used
[3] Objective and subjective social indicators used and related to each other

Most of the objective criteria used involved clinicians' judgments about normal functioning as the essential attribute of a higher QOL. It is difficult to judge whether there is any evidence to support this type of assessment by clinicians.

Table 3 shows the research designs and sampling of the studies. As you can see, most of them do not fulfill the requirement of standard statistical procedures.

Table 3
Research Design and Sampling Details of Studies Which Use QOL Criteria to Justify the Delivery of Health Care

\multicolumn{6}{Research design*}		
1	2	3	4	5	6	Sampling details	Sample size
				x**		Inadequate details provided	32
					x	Randomized	20-248
x						Random sample	95
x						Consecutive patients	50
x						All survivors	44
		x				No control of selection	190
x						No control of selection	17
			x			No control of selection	51
x						All survivors	18
				x**		Consecutive patients	200
x						All survivors	120
x						All survivors	19
			x			Consecutive patients	49
x**						Adequate sample of all treated patients	350

Research design*						Sampling details	Sample size
1	2	3	4	5	6		
x						Consecutive patients	55
x**						All treated patients	158
	x					Consecutive patients	20
		x**				Matched controls	62
x						Inadequate details provided	500
			x			Inadequate details provided	20
x						No control of self selection	10
x						Consecutive patients	51
x						Consecutive patients	10
14	2	2	2	2	1		

*Adapted from Campbell and Stanley
**Modified

[1] One-shot case study
[2] One group pretest/post-test design
[3] Static group comparison
[4] Non-equivalent control group design
[5] Time series
[6] Randomized clinical trial

If, on the other hand, one reviews the studies of psychosocial impact of breast cancer ignoring the term QOL, one finds a few statistically valid results.

Table 4 lists the most common and statistically well researched variables from the literature on breast cancer.

Table 4
Summary of the Variables Examined in the Psychological Literature on Breast Cancer and its Treatment

Psychosocial impact of breast cancer and its treatment
    Psychological discomfort
        Depression
        Anxiety
        Hostility
    Changes in life patterns
        Physical discomfort
        Marital/Sexual upset
        Activity level reduction/increase
    Fears and concerns
        Mastectomy/mutilation
        Cancer/death

Variables that influence intensity and duration of psychosocial impact

    Premorbid variables
        Patient characteristics
            Importance of physical appearance/breast to patient
            Age
            Preoperative expectations
        Environmental characteristics
            Preoperative preparation by surgeon
            Quality of marital/sexual relationship
    Post-mastectomy variables
        Patient coping styles
            Denial and related defenses
                (intensity and selectivity)
            Search for causes
                (self-blame and projection of blame)
    Environmental variable
        Time elapsed since surgery
        Availability of support
           (doctor/surgeon, spouse and family, and other patients)
        Additional medical treatments
           (radiotherapy and chemotherapy)

On the basis of larger projects such as Bahnson's studies in the 1960's (1964a, 1964b, 1965a, 1966, 1969), Weisman's Omega in the 1970's and later studies in the 1970's and 1980's, we can begin to select instruments which have been proven reliable and valid for our purposes.

If we can come to an agreement about the measurements to be used in the suggested common projects, the statisticians could select from the available models and the theories for the one that fits best.

References

Andrews, F. M., & Withey, S. B. *Social indicators of well-being.* New York: Plenum Press, 1976.

Bahnson, C. B., & Bahnson, M. B. Denial and repression of primitive impulses and of disturbing emotions in patients with malignant neoplasms. In D. M. Kissen, & L. LeShan (Eds.), *Psychosomatic aspects of neoplastic disease.* London: Pitman, 1964a.

Bahnson, C. B., and Bahnson, M. B. Cancer as an alternative to psychosis: a theoretical model of somatic and psychological regression. In D. M. Kissen, & L. LeShan (Eds.), *Psychosomatic aspects of neoplastic disease.* London: Pitman, 1964b.

Bahnson, C. B., & Bahnson, M. B. Ego defensive functioning in cancer patients. The utilization of denial and projection as measured by self-attributed and projected mood and emotion. Paper presented at the Fourth International Conference on Psychosomatic Aspects of Neoplastic Disease. Italy: Turin, 1965a.

Bahnson, C. B., & Bahnson, M. B. Role of the ego defenses: denial and repression in the etiology of malignant neoplasm. *Annals of the New York Academy of Sciences, 125,* 1966.

Bahnson, M. B., & Bahnson, C. B. Ego defenses in cancer patients. *Annals of the New York Academy of Sciences,* 1969, *164,* 335-343.

Blades, B. C. Quality of life after major burns. *Journal of Trauma*, 1979, *19*, 555-567.

Burt, R. S., Wiley, J. A., Minor, M. J., & Murray, J. R. Structure of well-being: form, content and stability over time. *Social Methods Research*, 1978, *6*, 365-407.

Campbell, A. P., Converse, P. E., & Rodgers, W. L. *The quality of American life.* New York: Russel Sage, 1976.

Campbell, D. T., & Stanley, J. C. *Experimental and quasi-experimental designs for research.* Chicago: Rand McNally, 1966.

Gerson, E. M. On "quality of life." *American Social Review*, 1976, *41*, 793-806.

Meyerowitz, B. E. Psychosocial correlates of breast cancer and its treatments. *Psychological Bulletin*, 1980, *87*, 108-131.

Najman, J. M., & Levine, S. Evaluating the impact of medical care and technologies on the quality of life. *Social Science Medicine*, 1981, *15*, 107-115.

Section II

❖

Life-Threatening Illness: Mind-Body Approaches and Psychotherapy

5

Working With AIDS Patients

Rudolph Klussmann, Thomas Baumann

By dealing with AIDS we are confronted with two problems that we usually tend to avoid: Sexuality and death. Furthermore, we experience once more helplessness regarding new diseases. This happens at a time where we believe that with the help of scientific progress we might control the world and perhaps human limitedness. Such a combination of death, sexuality and helplessness in connection with a disease has existed previously only during the centuries of syphilis.

Hence, this leads to a fear of the disease with feelings of helplessness, defenselessness and dependency. As for AIDS this fear consists of the following:

— The fear of infection by the enemy, i.e. the germ, as well as of the carrier who also becomes (part of) the enemy. Social rejection of the infected is the consequence, and his fear of being rejected is justified indeed.

— In HIV-positives there is in addition the fear of the outbreak of the disease. The uncertainty is considerably great, as no reliable figures are available showing how many HIV-positives succumb to the outbreak of the AIDS-syndrome.

— The fear of social isolation is particularly imminent in AIDS-patients, HIV-positives and presumed-infected individuals, conjuring mental diseases, venereal diseases, leprosy etc.

— Furthermore, one is reminded of archaic fears of an "artificial" disease caused by evil spirits or the devil. However, the loss of health and happiness is caused by external enemies (Klussmann, 1989).

In the following paragraphs I would like to point out some of the characteristics of the HIV-infection and the AIDS-syndrome:

— The biological course of the HIV-infection.
— The social groups of concern.
— The social dimension.

Particularities of the biological course of the HIV-infection

A patient's ability to handle the diagnosis HIV-positive and/or AIDS depends on both inner and outer factors. It seem essential to take account of these dual realities in the medical as well as in the psychotherapeutic practice. We have to consider both the clinical course of the disease, as well as the individuality of the patient and furthermore, the social environment and the attitudes of society in general.

From the psychoanalytical point of view the central trauma of the HIV-infected is the sudden realization of the loss of his invulnerability and integrity. Hence, the following questions arise: How does the AIDS-patient handle this trauma? What is his inner psychic defense like and how does it function? What are his compensating strategies and adaptive processes that he uses in order to defend himself from this offense (Weimer, Nilsson-Schonesson & Clement, 1989)?

The Ego is challenged in a number of different ways:

— Apart from having to cope with the above mentioned trauma it has to come to terms with intra-psychic conflicts that were well compensated for so far but might be reactivated. Such reactivated intra-psychic conflicts might be experienced as culpably experienced sexuality and feelings of guilt and shame.

— The fear of death will emerge with the same intensity as the fear of contamination in both afflicted and doctors/ psychotherapists alike. In particular, the transference of destructive thoughts endanger the doctor-patient-relationship, as will be discussed later (Bahnson, 1989).

The biological course of a HIV-infection can be divided into the following different phases: After an incubation period varying in length from patient to patient, a flu like illness occurs that will hardly be considered as a specific symptom. After a latency period lasting up to ten years or longer, the immune deficiency may become apparent with its related symptoms resulting now in an experienceable veritable disease. Now the life expectancy usually will span only over a period of months and death is certain.

On the background of such a schedule it becomes understandable that over a long period of the time, the afflicted have to live in considerable uncertainty. The very moment the test result HIV-positive is disclosed for the first time, has to be regarded as the predominant traumatic event in the patient's career; every follow-up test remains a continuous source of deadly menace. It has to be mentioned that this threat will be experienced as particulary distressing and may lead to depression, hypochondriac fears, and psychosomatic symptoms especially, since physical symptoms of the HIV-infection are often missing at this stage.

Consequently, in a number of cases the outbreak of AIDS results in psychological relief. One possible interpretation of this circumstance is the assumption that the patient regards the test results as foreign or external; whereas, the somatic disease with all its intrinsic destructive forces is experienced as internal, i.e. as a part belonging to the patient himself. When the diagnosis HIV-positive is disclosed, depressed and unconscious fantasies of death, guilt and punishment are activated and will be experienced as having become true. In the cases of the outbreak of the disease, the EGO is thus prepared. Fantasies become realities. Hence, the EGO is relieved.

As a result of the intensive exchange between psychosomatic medicine and psychoneuro-immunology, the question has emerged whether AIDS is a psychosomatic phenomenon that may be encountered by means of psychotherapy. Excessive hopes on the side of the patient towards the psychotherapist and perhaps on the side of the therapist himself, may result for the two of them in fantasies of omnipotence as well as magic and unrealistic expectations. Consequently, disappointment and aggressive conflicts are inevitable (Bahnson, 1989).

Particularities of the afflicted groups

In the following we will take a closer look at three main groups of the HIV-infected population:
— the homosexuals
— the hemophiliacs
— the i.v. drug-dependents

They have in common that during their former life they had to cope with numerous internal and external threats.

- For the homosexual the process of finding his own-self as well as the coming-out often is not completed. The need for emotions such as guilt, punishment and self reproachment are arduously compensated and might be reactivated by a HIV-positive diagnosis. This process might be more brisk, the more fragile the defense was, or the more conflictuous the (sexual) orientation has been so far.
- The bleeder carries a X-chromosomal inherited disease hence, the mother is the conductor. As a consequence, the mother develops guilt feelings for having mal-equipped her sons, which sometimes results in overprotective care. Furthermore, such a stigmatized son often means a hardly bearable mortification and offense for the father. He withdraws or denies and does not allow the son to progress out of the mother-child-dyad into autonomy. The process of psychological individuation

became easier when in the 1970's, self applicable coagulation factors suddenly were available.

However, in the 1980's, the threat of an HIV-infection resulting from the use of these factors jeopardized this possibility of an easier individuation. Hence the individuation process was subjected to a massive drawback resulting in regression towards the mother and reactivating pre-oedipal conflicts.

The defense of the handicap being the fear of helplessly bleeding to death, the defense of aggressive impulses, the arduously acquired identity, the dependency on the parents and the medical care system thus becomes apparent.

Another intra-psychic aspect of the bleeder has to be mentioned at this point: The medical doctors have successfully replaced the function of the "triangulating father" within the doctor-patient relationship. Thus they are fantasized as omnipotent objects, which (between 1980-1985) have applied contaminated blood preparations and therefore become death bringing "evil" fathers. Consequently, the helping alliance turns into a menacing relationship.

— The i.v. drug-dependent also were subjected to numerous traumatizations. Hence the HIV-infection threatens their laboriously erected and sustained defense formations. They are therefore particularly exposed to re-retraumatization.

It is worth taking into account that these three groups are dependent on the behaviour or the substance, which promotes the infection, i.e.:

— sexual behaviour

— coagulation factors and/or blood transfusions

— intravenously applied drugs

It is a remarkable characteristic that these dependencies are fantasized as good, pleasure spending objects which furthermore, are in the case of bleeders, life supporting. These very objects now bring about the deadly threat. As a result, fears of annihilation as experienced in early childhood are reactivated and might evoke defense mechanisms such as projective identification, splitting and denial. On the basis of these defense mechanisms it becomes understandable that destructive impulses in connection with the fear of annihilation leads to the fantasy of destroying (others) via infection. Such fantasies deriving from the unconscious are commonly being observed in our patients.

Furthermore, we observe fantasies of guilt arising from the idea that the HIV-infection has been acquired by personal behaviour, by own fault. According to Seidl (1991), these fantasies, which are close to consciousness, are used to ward off the feelings of helplessness and surrender in the face of the illness.

From a psychosomatic point of view, one may conclude that a predominant characteristic of AIDS is the following: The Ego (though marked by fear of annihilation, massive destructiveness and helplessness) does not disintegrate because it has the potential to fatally infect others. This (unconscious) fantasy protects the Ego from fragmentation. Hence, one has not observed a rise in suicides or suicide attempts as compared to other serious infectious diseases. In this context it should be underlined that the afflicted referred to above, are embedded in social networks in which they experience their own fate with others; on the other hand, they are confronted with the realization of their destructive fantasies against others.

Particularities of the social dimension

Particularly, the social environment of the AIDS-patient has to be taken into consideration: The accumulation of negative social reaction towards the illness, such as rejection, withdrawal and reproaches, adds to the general stigmatization of the afflicted groups of the homosexual, drug addicts and handicapped.

Therefore, fear of discrimination should not be interpreted exclusively as the defense mechanism of projection because of the nature of the social environment of each group, which provides a real background for these fears. This amalgamation of psychic defense mechanism and real discrimination can not easily be discerned by the interviewer/psychotherapist. The afflicted can not assume to be rewarded with a secondary gain of illness such as positive/empathetic attention of the society. Therefore, they attempt to conceal a HIV-positive diagnosis (Buchholz & Reich, 1987). From this derives the therapeutic difficulties. Hence, the therapist should always be aware of these dimensions of reality. He might be regarded as a representative of society and his counter-transference is endangered by slipping into the part of a pedagogue, a moralist or in contrary the role of an indignant critic of society. Thus, Freud's demand for an evenly suspended attention regains its specific meaning (Seidl, 1991).

The practice of AIDS counselling

On the background as outlined above, the authors would like to reflect in detail on the practice of AIDS-counselling for which we deem it necessary first to cite the following figures (Heusser, Bauer, Steiger & Gutzwiller, 1990):

— Counselling takes place with only 30-45% of all HIV-patients with risk prone behaviour.
— Prior to HIV-testing,General Practitioner's advise their patients in 88% of all cases; whereas, in the aftermath of such a test, only 27% of the patients have follow-up care.
— In only 33% of the patients a history of sexual behaviour is taken by the General Practitioner (GP), despite the fact that only 3% of the patients would be embarrassed by such inquiries.
— Almost all patients utilise the media as a source of specific information;whereas, less than half of them consult their GP. Furthermore, the patients regard only 12% of these consultations as particularly helpful.

— The means for patient information are insufficient in most medical offices:
In the Anglo/American countries, handouts are available in about 50% of all medical offices; however, in Switzerland handouts are rarely seen in any office at all, and slogans such as "a medical office is not a place for prevention" are advocated.

The main handicaps for HIV-preventive work in medical offices are the following:

— Only 50% of the doctors feel sufficiently competent.
— Inhibitions on the side of the doctor to talk about sexuality.
— Prejudices against homosexuals, drug addicts (and handicapped).
— The doctors' fear of an infection of himself and/or of one of his other patients.
— The priority of curative medicine to preventive medicine.

Counselling of HIV-patients is of special importance as there is no curative therapy available at the present time. Usually the reason for a consultation lies in symptoms of fear and depression as well as in real social discrimination. With the progression of the disease then, arise problems such as social isolation; helplessness and hopelessness; and dealing with death and dying.

The doctor or therapist must consider a number of different aspects of the patient including: the present state of the disease (i.e. HIV-positive test result, lymphocyte count, manifestation of the syndrome); the psychological situation of the patient, i.e. symptoms, coping strategies, social integration; present attitudes towards the illness (ex. risk prone behaviour towards self or others).

Specific problems arise during the HIV-test counselling which could be partially avoided if the following conditions were met:

— The indication for the test ought to be strictly on behalf of medical reasons.

— The patient's consent should be a prerequisite to the test as well as an opportunity to gain information concerning preventive measures.

— The patients personal circumstances should be elucidated.

The potential *advantages* of the combination of HIV-testing plus counselling cannot be overlooked. Some of these advantages are:

— Making a diagnosis
— Providing better care (secondary prevention, early therapy)
— Reducing unwarranted fears
— Providing a motivation to change behavioral patterns, including adding the element of certainty as a precondition for cognitive processes.
— Providing helpful information for decision making using information derived from sexual practices, attitude towards the partner, attitude towards the use of (illegal) drugs, occuptational plans (as well as financial obligations etc.)

The potential *disadvantages* of an HIV-test include psychological reactions; stigmatization and isolation promoted by partners and/or close persons, and the professional environment; possible uncontrolled data-transmission; and in the case of an HIV-negative result, the development of an unjustified feeling of security.

Check-list for counselling of a patient *prior* to an HIV-test:

— Reasons for the test
— Risk prone behaviour and risk situations
— Check knowledge about the transmission of HIV and means of prevention
— Discuss advantages and disadvantage of HIV-testing
— Possible consequences (positive as well as negative) of the HIV-test result concerning:

Working With AIDS Patients

- Psychic reactions
- Sexual relationships
- Drug consuming behaviour
- Occupational/professional situation
- Medical care
- Health insurance

— When and in which way will the test result be communicated?
— Protection of sexual partners
— Social network of the patient:

- Person of confidence
- Contacts/friends while waiting for the test result

— Arrange a date for the next consultation/appointment
— Advise where to seek help in case that problems occur

Checklist for counselling of the patient *in the aftermath* of an HIV-test:

— Inform the client of the result
— Does the client understand what the result means?
— In the case of a negative result:

- Stress the importance of preventive measures (in order to stay negative)
- Retesting after three months time (only if necessary)

— In the case of a positive result:

- Who shall be informed and in what way?
- What does the client plan to do during the following hours and days?
- Where does the client see the main difficulties?
- Discuss preventive measures.
- Assure the client that strong emotional reaction to his new situation are common.
- Inform about the possibility of consulting an AIDS-

ambulance or a self-help group (e.g. AIDS-Hilfe).
- Discuss further steps of medical care.
- Transfer to a specialist if necessary.
- Arrange further appointments to monitor psychological development and reactions.
- Specify where the client may turn to in case of an emergency (Heusser et. al, 1990).

The best way to prevent panic actions is by providing comprehensive information to the patient during the counselling, prior to an HIV-test on the basis of a well established doctor-patient relationship. Almost a third of those which want to be tested are afraid of an infection but do not belong to a (high) risk group. Sometimes such fears are manageable by comprehensive information. However, in other cases these fears are part of an AIDS-phobia as a feature of a neurotic personality.

Given an HIV-positive diagnosis the psychosocial counselling is predominantly directed towards psychological coping strategies. Based on our own counselling experience as well as on the expertise of others, the following topics turn out to be most important:

1) The *communication of information* by which means lack of knowledge can be compensated, fears be diminished and hence, the attitude towards the infection be improved.

2) Depression, anxiety and suicidal tendencies are common reactions that are linked to guilt feelings and fear of social isolation. During *crisis intervention* the consultant/doctor should be aware of these feelings and accept them as such. If possible they should be discussed with the patient.

3) The HIV-patient has to forgo his usual *sexual behaviour* in order to protect himself and/or his partner. Such a renunciation requests work of mourning. Furthermore, one's own desires and emotions are experienced as

threatening. Consequently, the self acceptance will be rendered unstableresulting in further impairment of a positive attitude towards life, which might require therapeutic intervention.

4) Since sometimes job and/or housing might be jeopardized additional problems in coping can arise with the disease. Financial as well as legal aid should be made available.

The difficulties in counselling HIV-patients stems from having to accept on the one hand, emotions such as anxiety, rage, and depression, but on the other hand to convey an attitude of a positive orientation towards the future. Drug addicts should be motivated to contact self-help groups and/or AIDS-ambulances where both problems i.e. drug dependency as well as an additional HIV-infection are taken into consideration.

Transference and counter-transference in dealing with AIDS-patients

In order to deal adequately with HIV-positive results, matters concerning transference as well as counter transference become particularly important. The experience derived from psychotherapeutic and psychoanalytic treatment during interviews or patient counselling should be exploited for the benefit of patients and doctors. We have to be aware that the therapeutic process and its transference mechanisms depend on the development of the somatic disease. It is always a treatment "in the face of the death".

The mechanism of transference is predominantly of a narcissistic nature. The desire to participate and to merge with a health omnipotent object. The diagnosis HIV-positive usually causes a shock, a severe narcissistic crisis. Due to the loss of invulnerability, the Ego is confronted with overwhelming destructive fantasies, as well as with these destructive fantasies coming true. By offering this type of transference the therapist is experienced as an ideal (self) object. Thus, hopes arise of recompensation as well as restoration of the endangered physical and psychological identity. Simultaneously, aggressive and destructive impulses will be transferred as well.

Thus one might interpret the situation in the following way: that the afflicted wants to survive or die with the therapist. Rage, aggression and envy all directed against the therapist are found alongside with the desire to preserve him as a good and healthy object (Weinel, 1989).

We should not forget that the therapist frequently will be regarded as a representative/executive of the health care system and of the society as well. Hence it becomes understandable that fears of discrimination and persecution are always present and may lead to distrust and hostility. Frequently, counter-transference will be raised as a result of the offered type of transference feelings of omnipotence.The therapist believes he/she is able to influence the course of the disease. Feelings of might, as well as helplessness, bring about an oscillation between guilt feelings, because he survives and feelings of integrity and immunity. Furthermore, feelings of inadequacy and futility may result in pronounced counter-transference resistance. Consequently empathy towards the patient is markedly reduced. The high degree of expectancy on the patient's side weighs on the therapist. He tries to get rid of the burden by keeping his distance (The German language uses the idiom: "Sich jemanden vom Leibe halten." To keep away someone's body.) with the aim quickly to get rid of the patient.

At the bottom of this psychodynamic mechanism, frequently fears of contamination are observed as well as unsolved conflicts regarding sexuality and death. Hence the therapeutic process is endangered since the therapist is not available as a transference object. He losses the immediate contact to the unconscious processes, because he defends his own regressive tendencies which correspond with those of the patient. For example instead of analyzing his own fears, he intellectualizes or feels board. Alternatively he might (re)act as directed by the patient's transference rather than reflecting his counter-transference in order to achieve a basis for therapeutic intervention (Adler & Beckett, 1989).

Problems with counter-transference and counter-transference resistance might become apparent by the following behavioral pattern:

— To lay precipitate emphasis onto reality.
— To convert feelings of omnipotent into promises of being able to heal and help.
— To identify with the patient and thus hinder his work of mourning.
— To suffer with the patient instead of offering understanding and company.

Therefore, occasionally the contact with AIDS-patients results in impressive and sometimes irrational reactions on the side of the consultant. For example, after an one-hour interview with an depressive HIV-positive patient, the author noticed that he subjected himself to an act of quickly washing his hands knowing that an infection was impossible.

Even more impressive seems the report of an empathetic medical student: She admitted that she always had great problems to deal with AIDS-patients due to her fear of infection. But even more important would be the fear that someone else would become aware of her fear. One day she took an elevator together with a slim young man whom she considered to be an AIDS-patient. A feeling of panic arose in her with numb feet and tickling fingers. In the same night she had the following dream:" Standing under a tin roof I observe a distant nuclear power plant, which however seems to be very close. The slim young man who was in the elevator yesterday is sitting at the switchboard. He is connected to the power plant with a cannula and his blood flows into the reactor. I am afraid that the whole thing blows up - and I wake up". The brief comment of the student:" To me this means total destruction".

By managing HIV-infection and AIDS, the horrible, helpless and hopeless feeling emerges of how to handle all these problems. However, I like to point out that AIDS as well as any other disease, contains a potential to build up psychological structures and to be supportive in reorganizing and/or organizing a new inner and outer reality in the sense of an individuation process. Real work of mourning may mobilize energies to define new aim and to build up new relationships.

To conclude, We would like to use the analogy to the cancer in Greek mythology: When Hercules fought the hydra he was bitten by a cancer. As a reward for the cancer who supported the hydra in her strife against Hercules, Hera the mother of gods raises the cancer to the firmament, as a sign of the zodiac and places him next to the lion. According to Kerenyi, it is within the sign of the cancer where the human soul descends into lower regions, and it is here where the underworld half of heaven begins. According to the myth we may assume that the cancer belongs to the realm of the evil, the Hades. He hides in the struggle against the dark powers. He tries to block the way to one's self and thus the way into autonomy and individuation. But the antimony also becomes apparent. Hercules (the Greek Herakles is "the one Hera gave the glory") has to fight and to overpower the evil to find himself. The cancer renders the fight even more difficult and is therefore rewarded by becoming a sign of the zodiac.

Beside the negative aspect of the evil " swallowing" mother, there is the positive one which drives the son to his deeds to his process of individuation. Also in the psychology of the zodiac the cancer marks the reflection of the emotional feelings at a turning point: Passing the climax, the further descent is lined out and marks the end of our being. "Our fate is destined by the stars",but does that include the cancer as well? Anyhow, man has matured when he is able to accept his fate:

— To be defeated

— To become ill

— To die (Klussmann, 1990)

The sprawling cancer-disease as well as the progression of the AIDS-disease limits our grandiose self. Maybe the myth ought to tell us that from this point of view, the paradox has to be understood: That the illness is interpreted as a first step towards the establishment of health.

Acknowledgement

We would like to thank D.P.Wichelhaus for the translation of this article into the English language and for secretarial work.

References

Adler, G., & Beckett, A. Psychotherapy of the patient with an HIV Infection: some ethical and therapeutic dilemmas. *Psychosomatics*, 1989, *30*, 203-208.
Bahnson, C.B. Psychodynamischer Zugang zum AIDS-Kranken. Psychosomatische und psychotherapeutische Aspekte. In (Hrsg. R. Klussmann, F.-D. Goebel): *Psychosomatische Medizin im interdisziplinären terdisziplinären Gespräch: Zur Klinik und Praxis der AIDS-Krankheit.* Springer, New York, 1989, 25-31.
Buchholz, M.B. & Reich, G. Panik, Panikbedarf, Panikverarbeitung. Soziopsychoanalytische Anmerkungen zu zeitgenössischen Integratinsprozessen aus Anlass von Tschernobyl und AIDS. *Psyche*, Stuttgart, 1987, 610-639.
Heusser, R., Bauer, G. Steiger, Th.S., & Gutzwiller, F. AIDS-Beratung in der Praxis. *Therapeutische Umschau*, Bern, *47*, 1990, 741-748.
Klussmann, R. Vom Umgang mit den AIDS-Kranken und der AIDS-Krankheit. In (Hrsg. R. Klussmann, F.-D.Goebel): *Psychosomatische Medizin im interdisziplinären Gespräch: Zur Klinik und Praxis der AIDS-Krankheit*, Springer, New York,1989, 61-66.
Klussmann, R. zur Bedeutung des Wortes "Krebs" im täglichen Sprachgebrauch, in der Mythologie, im Traum In (Hrsg R. Klussmann, B. Emmerich): *Psychosomatische Medizin im interdisziplinären Gespräch: Der Krebskranke*, Springer, New York, 1990, 3-6.
Seidl, O. Psychosoziale Forschung und Therapie mit HIV-Infizierten, *Psychosozial*, 1991, *14*, 33-42.
Weimer, E., Nilsson-Schonesson, L., & Clement, U. HIV-

Infektion: Trauma und Traumaverarbeitung, *Psyche*, 1989, Stuttgart, *43*, 720-735.

Weinel, E., Überlegungen zu Übertragungs-und Gegenübertragungs-reaktionen bei der Behandlung von AIDS-Patienten, *Psyche*, Stuttgart, *43*, 710-719.

6

Ethical Issues in Psychotherapy With Cancer Patients

Thomas Küchler

Introduction

Article 1 of the German Constitution begins with the words: "The dignity of a human being is unimpeachable." This ethical principle stands in clear contrast to everyday reality for many cancer patients suffering from the effects of their disease as well as the effects of therapy, to such an extent that the question of human dignity is posed anew for them every single day. Although this question of dignity primarily pertains to ethics in somatic medicine, psychotherapy will have to take a stand on ethical questions along with its growing involvement with cancer patients.

In these times of computerized search for literature it takes no great effort to conclude that among the approximately 380,000 publications dealing with cancer published from 1980 to the present, there is not one volume dealing with the concepts of ethics, psychotherapy and cancer combined in one title. This is all the more surprising since everyone concerned with cancer patients in psychotherapy in one way or another is confronted with these problems, be they only latent. In view of the lack of primary references on the one hand and the variety of general ethical codes on the other, this contribution, which is primarily based on practical observations, can only be considered as a first draft and impetus to discussion.

Psychotherapeutic Interventions With Cancer Patients

In psychotherapy with cancer patients there are two basically different settings to be considered: first, care in acute phases, generally taking place within the medical institution, such as the hospital, out-patient clinic, and oncological practice (von Kerekjarto, 1986; Ratsak, 1986). Secondly, "regular" psychotherapy is usually found outside of primarily caretaking institutions, that is, in the therapist's office, health centers and outpatient departments. The basic principles for psychotherapy in these two areas may well be identical, yet there are specific problems which demand separate consideration. The most common forms of psychotherapeutic intervention are—depending on the kind of disease and the setting—supportive therapy, crisis intervention, biographically oriented methods based on Gestalt-therapy, especially the life-panorama technique and family consultation therapy.

In the following the author will limit his discussion to two main themes. One will be general ethical principles in psychotherapy for cancer patients, the other specific problems in this field which are resistant to simple solutions.

General Ethical Principles

The author's personal set of values acquired during his training and work as a gestalt therapist is in the main identical with the values that are fundamental to medicine based on ethics: I always try to respect and strengthen my patients' AUTONOMY, that is, their freedom to make their own decisions. I try to use my knowledge and abilities in the best interest of my patients; this includes becoming acquainted with medical therapy methods and the findings of psycho-oncological research beyond my fundamental knowledge as a psychotherapist (BENEVOLENCE). I attempt, as far as possible, to be aware of the scope of manipulative possibilities inherent in the techniques of psychotherapy and examine my interventions for their possible detrimental effects (such as breaking down a patient's defenses, or projecting personal interests). This law of NIHIL-NOCERE also includes taking into account the emotional participation of relatives even beyond the death of the patient. I will try not to discriminate against a patient for reasons of sympathy, special scientific interest, age or sex (JUSTICE). I strive for TRUTHFULNESS (this may not be equated with brutal openness). I consider all communications of my patients confidential as a matter of principle and only pass information on to medical staff with their consent and am aware at all times of the RESPONSIBILITY I have as psychotherapist within the entire therapeutic team.

Hope, Fear and Repression

This set of values, perhaps idealistic, is often threatened in therapy with cancer patients, for a variety of reasons. This may be clarified by two examples:

An 18-year old patient suffering from Ewing sarcoma has had chemotherapy with no success. The only way to prolong his life expectancy—prolonging in this case means several weeks—is carrying through a hemi-pelvectomy, i.e., amputation of a leg and parts of the pelvis. The surgeon is in favor of this measure and pleads for it with conviction and commitment; the oncological internist is of the opinion that the boy should be allowed to die in peace. Both can justifiably appeal to ethical considerations, and both have secondary motivations, which cannot be discussed here since they can only be guessed at. Asked for advisory support the author finds a young man who, in spite of his enormous swollen leg, is in high spirits because he has just learned that no metastases in the lung can be found. He refuses the amputation of the leg, telling me that he fears it may lead to impotence. "That business with the leg is definitely lousy," but he wants to have children some day. Careful questioning brings no evidence that he realizes that his death is imminent within the next few days or weeks and that these last days of his life without an operation may be the worst time a person can possibly imagine. The question of how a responsible therapist guided by ethics ought to deal with such a situation will have to be left unanswered at this point as well as in my second example:

A 42-year old woman with a degree in pharmacology but showing very little self-confidence in the beginning is suffering from metastases in the bones after a primary breast cancer and in the course of ambulant therapy reports her wish to consult a diviner. She wants him to advise her in rearranging her apartment to make sure that the furniture, especially the beds, do not stand in the path of negative rays. The woman is in psychotherapy, takes hormone therapy prescribed by the oncological internist and regularly visits a non-medical practitioner. During the last year no new metastases were found and the patient seems to be on her way to being cured at this point.

Suffering in Guilt Turns into Fighting for Life

This second example differs from the first in more than one aspect: The situation is not that of a first consulting interview but a therapy setting with mutual knowledge of possible developments in the long run. Even if a diviner has no place in the author's personal set of values, he understands fully well the diviner's importance for the patient. There is always a necessity to introduce a little magic into the highly technical routine of cancer treatment and most psycho-oncological research results show that active, non-compliant patients with fighting potential show the most favorable prognosis as far as mortality rate is concerned (Rogentine, 1979). Yet it is especially here that we see the chance to come to terms with the basic fears that accompany the outbreak of cancer without endangering defense structures. However, there is another difficult matter showing up in this patient and her way of dealing with the disease: Behind the concept of "I-must-try-out-anything" there is often the notion that the disease itself or not getting better is somehow one's own fault. The psychotherapist who accepts the patient's desire for analysis or biographical work uncritically may tend to overlook the latent masochism behind this wish, the desire to find the final proof of one's own guilt in the process of becoming sick (Becker, 1986).

On the other hand working on the biography of a patient may well provide the chance to overcome this element of guilt and so turn the casual everyday self-punishments—be they large or small—of so many cancer patients into active autonomous desires for life.

The Threat to Autonomy

Our first example shows, on the other hand, how far the autonomy of a patient can be restricted without any indication of whether this is detrimental or favorable for him. The author's conflict in such a situation has to do primarily with a basic decision: Is it possible for the patient (in keeping with the principle of NIHIL-NOCERE, mentioned above) to discuss his defense mechanisms within the minimal amount of time available to realistically view the short span of time remaining to him, and does he personally have enough energy and time to go about this together with the patient if it is at all possible. In this situation (a first consultative interview) I decided that this was not possible and attempted to secure psychological care in his home town in case he or his relatives might want to take advantage of this assistance. This decision seemed to have been the right one in retrospect as well. However, bewilderment and shock remained concerning the young man and his fate and the helpless state into which the disease put all those concerned.

This example may well seem a bit extraordinary in many respects; yet it is not altogether atypical, at least as far as the strong restriction of personal responsibility in making decisions is concerned. Of all the values that ideally govern the actions of the psychotherapist, personal autonomy of the patient definitely ranks highest. For cancer patients this autonomy, i.e., the capacity to make personal decisions in a responsible manner, may be restricted for different reasons:

1. Lack of access to all relevant facts necessary for making a decision. The vital necessity of adequate information is at stake here as it always is. Although it is now the rule to inform the patient of all the essential facts, legal considerations often seem to influence the course of the doctor-patient discussions. Whether the patient has been able to take in the given information to the point of making an autonomous decision based on it will depend mainly on the emotional commitment of the practitioner in charge.
2. Vital defense mechanisms. These defenses, especially in the case of patients faced with death, may change in manner, degree and intensity from one day to the next, sometimes from one hour to the next (Bahnson, 1982);
3. The family situation. Especially in new and frightening situations, well-known patterns of denial and the wish to protect are favored out of fear over open and emotional communication strategies. No relative dares touch the topics felt to be taboo in such cases (Bahnson, 1979).
4. The socially-enforced attitude which allows us to complain about "those doctors." On the other hand, this attitude does not tolerate acts of real revolt, for example, refusing a proposed treatment.
5. Religiously determined values. These values may consider sickness as fate, punishment or trial, etc., and therefore beyond the patient's active, autonomous influence.

The greatest impediment to the autonomy of the patient is, however, the indispensable medical expertise necessary for decision-making. Highly specialized familiarity with chemotherapy, with intensities of radiation and surgical practice, leads necessarily to the patient's trustfully abandoning himself to the appropriate treatment—behavior which the literature refers to as regression and heaps into the category "defense mechanisms"—or else to submit to treatment with fear and reluctance. The ideal, of course, is informed consent.

Personal Fears of the Psychotherapist

The most important task for the psychotherapist working with cancer patients is to support or to repair this severely threatened autonomy of the patient. This calls for a comparably strong autonomy on the part of the psychotherapist himself. This therapeutic autonomy is quite naturally similarly threatened, especially since the therapist is confronted with his or her own fear of dying. Every cancer patient is confronting us with death, his death and our own death. My personal attitude towards the limitedness of life, my personal consciousness about the meaning of my own life now and in the future (Petzold, 1984), and a personal attitude toward making a conscious effort not to make use of my defense mechanisms, but to recognize them as such, all of these add up to make a therapist's capability to hear those thoughts and emotions the cancer patient is unable or reluctant to express to other persons. In short, for ethical, and certainly not for formal educational reasons, a therapist ought to be confronted with his or her own fears of dying in the course of training and work with cancer patients.

Now the general idea is not to make the impression that working with oncological patients focuses mainly on death, quite the contrary. But only a person realizing the impact of the presence of death can be free for life. The appropriate way of dealing with an anus praeter, the enjoyment of a good meal, memories of long times past showing up when sleep refuses to come, a certain new (old) insecurity in sexual matters, a personal relationship to the creator of all things, in short the entire variety of life suddenly seen under different aspects may now be thought about and discussed.

At the same time there is a general difficulty. These thoughts will be interrupted time and again by moments of despair, depression and hopelessness. Whether the patient is shrinking away from the topic at hand or is reacting in an adequate manner is not always easy to decide.

Denial and Truth

Summarizing, I shall now refer once more to the validating terms of "TRUTH," "BENEVOLENCE" and "NIHIL-NOCERE." E. Kubler-Ross pointed out the different phases of accepting death as a final process, as early as 1969. A theory introducing phases of this structure can only provide an approximation for each individual case in accepting the inevitable. Many patients only show a few of the phases described. Although the model seems to be of restricted validity, most patients do deny the disease and its consequences for some time; hardly any patient denies it continually. Signs of the present emotional state of mind can be more often found in nonverbal than in verbal messages of the patient (Kuchler, 1986). By supporting this denial for a certain time I act according to the principle of NIHIL-NOCERE, if I am convinced that the attitude of the patient in question is in accordance with his healthy defense mechanisms (Kuchler, 1982). Such a procedure is in conflict with my commitment to truthfulness, only if I maintain this denial on my own, regardless of the actual process. This may happen, as mentioned before, when my own fears are pushed into the foreground, or if I have become so psychologically exhausted that I fear that I will be incapable of bearing the usually rather strong emotions that follow after defense has been abandoned. I have often met with this emotional fatigue in people working with cancer patients and I consider it natural. Nobody can be occupied primarily with pain and sorrow without suffering from "contagion" after a while, without being damaged himself or at least diminishing his reserves of uninhibited enjoyment of life. Therefore I think it is necessary for a psychotherapist to participate in a regular form of supervision—with special focus on the process of delimitation and confluence—as well as to have a solid network of colleagues, relatives and friends he can rely on. The lone ranger in the field of psychotherapy with cancer patients is harmful. For in addition to professional competence, which is to be taken for granted, it is especially the capability for enjoyment which is fundamental to fulfilling the ethical commandment of benevolence.

References

Bahnson, C. B. Dying, death and the family. *Interaction 2*, 1979, 155-164.
Bahnson, C. B. Psychosomatic issues in cancer. In Gallon (Ed.), *The psychosomatic approach to illness*. New York: Elsevier North Holland, 1982.
Becker, H. Psychoonkologie. Heidelberg: Springer, 1986.
von Kerekjarto, M. U. S. Schug (Hrsg.), *Psychosoziale Betreuung von Tumorpatienten im ambulanten und stationären Bereich*. München: Zuckschwert, 1987.
Kübler-Ross, E. *On death and dying*. New York: Macmillan, 1969.
Küchler, Th. Die Angst, keine Antwort zu haben. *Z. f. humanistische psychologie*, 1/2, 1982.
Küchler, Th. Nonverbale Kommunikation bei Krebspatienten. Vortrag auf dem 18. Deutschen Krebskongress in München, 1986.
Petzold, H. Vorüberlegungen und Konzepte zu einer integrativen Persönlichkeitstheorie. *Z. f. Integrative Therapie*, 1/2, 1984, 73-115.
Ratsak, G. Die psychosoziale Betreuung von Krebspatienten in der Akutphase. Vortrag im Rahmen des 30-jahrigen Bestehens der Genesendenhilfe, 1986.
Rogentine, G. M. Psychological factors in the prognosis of malignant melanoma: a prospective study. *Psychosomatic Medicine*, 1979, *41*, 647-655.

7

Encouragement of the Incurably Ill

Hans Peter Bilek

Patients who seek psychotherapy always do so in despair. Their life situation looks hopeless to them; there is no perspective to a solution. Incurably ill and dying persons experience the threat of death, especially along the occidental patterns of self interpretation, as a catastrophy and self-destroying event. It is one of our most important concerns to face disease and death in a way that does not exclude human dignity. The task of psychotherapy is to encourage persons to find this way. This encouragement is therefore a central concern in many different therapeutic approaches.

This chapter elaborates on the question of encouragement in connection with severe disease or in the phase of dying, where it is as necessary as it is difficult. It is in the extreme situations of human life where our true problems crystallize; and this is where the psychotherapist can learn about the basic difficulties of life of his patients. In the following I shall try to show that human experiences, from biblical times until modern depth psychology, have a common denominator which consists of coping with the fact of our own incarnation; this includes our mortality.

Closer observation of the title shows that it contains a contradiction: Those who let themselves be encouraged are no more incurable. The old joke of the enuretic and his psychiatrist can explain that more clearly: The enuretic is asked

Encouragement of the Incurably Ill

whether psychotherapy has helped, and answers "yes." "So you don't urinate in bed anymore?"—"Yes I do," is the answer, "but I don't mind anymore." For the sake of the joke, the rest of the story is skipped: The symptom most likely disappeared at the moment in which the person didn't mind, because at the moment where he masters his shame, the symptom loses its function.

It is quite evident that the phenomenon of courage has always been on the human mind. Pericles says: "Be sure that the secret of happiness is freedom, but the secret of freedom is courage." As Dreikurs (1981) emphasizes, encouragement is an art that cannot be learned and trained mechanically. And Alice Miller (1981) gives an answer to the question where courage comes from: She suggests that Jesus Christ's courage to go his way is based on the experience of a self that has been enforced by love and understanding from his father Joseph.

The concept of cure is related to the concept of salvation. The former comes from a medical, the latter from a religious context. But especially in cases where medicine proves to be inefficient and declares patients to be incurable, the question arises to which extent an inability to cure somebody becomes equivalent with the inability to save him. Wherever a relation between the notions of cure and of salvation can be assumed, such a relation suggests that they both contain some of the hope for totality, complexity, and completeness.

In the bible dictionary, the notion of salvation is defined as "liberation from different kinds of distress" (Bibeltheologisches Woerterbuch). In the Greek bible, the notion of salvation is synonymous to the following notions: Escape, Save, Rescue, Let loose, Let live (notions of this type have been mentioned repeatedly by cancer patients; either directly, or in some disguised form). On the other hand, the incurable are the main body of clients for psychotherapists; and especially those doctors who are oriented towards depth-psychology base their hopes on Freud's experiences that opening the view for a new dimension in therapy opens chances for a cure, and thereby start from the assumption that even in moments where there is no solution available, the unconscious is a source of new chances for cure. This is how the extent becomes visible to which the findings of depth psychology relate to archaic imaginations.

Using a case report I want to show how the diagnosis of incurability can originate, and which alternatives can appear. The patient was 54 years old, his father was Jewish. According to his report, this was unknown to his family until the Nazis required the proof of ancestry. It was proposed to the then 17-year-old to volunteer for the German army because of his descendence. He participated in the invasion of Normandy, became a French prisoner, and evaded starvation by volunteering to become a French legionary. He went to Vietnam and was present in Dien Bien Phu. Back in Austria, he married a woman 10 years his senior. They ran a coal-store together. Both in 1979 and 1981 the patient had a cardiac infarction and was twice clinically dead. Later he developed paroxysms that were primarily mistaken as Adams-Stokes type. When it later turned out there were no ECG-changes during these paroxysms, the somatic treatment by the internal disease therapist became considerably less enthusiastic.

He was labeled "incurable" and transferred to a psychosomatic ward. In the course of the therapy it turned out that he, who used to carry 100 lbs of coal to the fourth floor every day, felt totally worthless, now that he was no more physically able to do these things. It was this feeling which also caused several attempts of suicide during the beginning of therapy. Encouragement to live in a new world of values made him recover, with the exception of his reduced heart capacity.

This case example, and psychosomatic experiences, unravel a frequent mistake in medicine: Loss of seemingly or actually irreplaceable bodily functions is equated with incurability. Most often, "incurable" means in medicine that the patient will die from his disease. But dying is not a disease. Dying is the irrevocable consequence of our being incarnated. For being irrevocable, all that remains is the question of HOW to die. This is where the difficulty of the topic appears again: When somebody is in an incurable somatic state, which is often the case in cancer patients, then the only logical therapeutic action is encouragement to death. But how is that to happen? There can be no doubt that our readiness to accept death is influenced by the image which we have of death. And it is exactly the occidental Christian myth which raises horror, if we think of the picture of the mower, the scythe man, and also of the tortures which Jesus Christ had to suffer until resurrection.

In this apparent discrepancy between "having to" die on one hand, and being confronted with an image of death whose threatening tradition is thousands of years old, I went out to search for alternatives. In some areas I was successful. First, a report by Hollos (1946), a Hungarian psychoanalyst, on his experiences of an extermination during World War II.

> A significant change must have taken place in my ego, by which a certain highest danger lost its weight. The change of ego served as a defense against the unbearably painful. I can recall very exactly how I made a turn, precipitated with my ego, almost with the feeling in my body. But it lasted for a second, and it lasted for eternity. In this sudden downfall of my ego I was at the same time dizzy and bright, and made a sudden, but fundamental account with my life, and without any idea of how that happened, silence came over my mind. More and more, like an enchanting discovery, silence overwhelmed me. I have come to terms, with no sign of disgust I go this last earthly way. Today I cannot imagine this peacefulness, nor explain it. By that time, we must have been in a state where heaven opened towards us.

The second contribution comes from a book in which the well-known international mountain climber Reinhold Messner (1978) has collected reports from persons who once had fallen in the mountains and had survived.

> Klaus Mohrmann has fallen: My fall was in the west flank of the "grosses Seehorn." We went on blank ice,

one step broke out, I fell. First, no thoughts, no fear. I hoped that my companion H. would be able to hold me and just tried to slow my ride down by pressing down the pickaxe. But my fall pulled H. away from his position. Now I knew: It's serious! I became totally purposeful and tried to hit the pickaxe into the ice with my hand. Finally, after repeated trials, it grasped, and I got hold. In the same moment I saw my companion rush down, at my left. But I was unable to notice his position. I was totally calm. I released the pickaxe with one hand, to get hold of the running rope. With the other hand I held on to the pickaxe in the ice. I was afraid of the heavy rope-tension and wanted to absorb it a little by the elasticity of my bent arm. My whole concentration focused on this activity. Also, I was totally convinced of my success. But when the rope stretched, I was pulled down in that very moment. The pickaxe flipped out of my hand, I precipitated and rushed down, head first. There were no thoughts, instinctively I threw myself on my belly and tried to slow the crazy ride down by pushing my hands forward; which was in vain on the blank ice. Having gotten such a strong pull, my speed was higher than the one of my friend, so I caught up. Again, an instinctive action: I pushed H. with all my strength towards his shoulders and threw him out of his track. This had hardly happened when I saw the cleft appear ahead of me. Before, I had not been thinking of it seriously, although we had crossed it. I had hoped we would land safely on the flat part of the glacier. Now I realized the hopelessness of any rescue, and in that same moment a feeling of relief came over me. Like in a flash, I saw the "kleine Seehörner" across, then a very colorful picture, of which I recall just the existence, but not its quality. But it was not me who saw, felt, and experienced this, but a second ego outside myself, that now watched the rushing body from a higher viewpoint. Then came the crack. Between the moment of realization of the end and the crack, according to later reconstruction, there must have been only a few seconds with about 40 meters of downfall, because the cleft could not be seen. But still, they appeared to me an eternity, which nevertheless was filled up with feelings of perfect happiness. I felt as if I had no essence. The crash itself felt like a sudden stop, disagreeable because there was no transition at all, but without any pain. I just said a relieving "Thank God" to myself, and then fainted.

These were two reports of men who went to the very border, and one can see that life in this area seems to follow other rules. A third example of "how it could be" can be found in Leo Tolstoi (1981), who describes his last phase in his novel, *The Death of Ivan Illich* (translated by the author):

Yes, all this was not the very true, he said to himself. But this does not matter. One can still achieve it, the very true. But what is the very true, he asked himself, and suddenly became all quiet. This happened towards the end of the third day, two hours before his death. Around the same time, the little schoolboy had secretly sneaked in, to his father, and approached his bed. The dying man still shouted and threw his hands around, in despair. His hand happened to land on his son's head. The little schoolboy grasped it, pressed it towards his lips, and started to cry. And at the same time it happened that Ivan Illich felt himself precipitate, and saw the light, and it became clear to him that his life had not been the very true; that it should have been, and that this could still be achieved. He had asked himself what the very true was, and had become silent, and listened. There he felt how somebody kissed his hand. He opened his eyes and looked at his son. He felt pity for him. His wife approached. He looked at her, too. With open mouth she stood there, her nose and cheeks covered by tears, and her face looked so desperate. And for her, too, he felt pity, so much pity. Yes, I am torturing her, it went through his mind. They feel harm. But it will be easier for them when I will have died. He wanted to express this thought, but was no more able. Why talk, by the way. One has to do it; he pondered. With one glance he drove his wife's attention to his son and said: "continue . . ., very sorry . . ., you, too." He wanted to add "farewell," but his tongue slipped, and since he was no more able to correct himself, he could only make a weak gesture with his hand, knowing that who was to understand would understand. And all of a sudden it became clear to him that everything that had tortured him and would not come out, that all these things suddenly and at once started floating out; from two sides, from ten sides, from all sides. He pitied those, and now it had to happen so that they would feel no more harm. Free them, and free himself of this harm. How good and how simple, he thought. And where is the pain, he asked himself; where has it gone. Tell me, where have you gone, pain. And he started listening. Oh, that's where it is. What does this matter, let it be pain. And death, where is it? And he looked for his fear of death, he had been so used to, and could not find it. Where was it? And what death? There was no anxiety, since there wasn't any death either. Instead of death there was a light. "That's what it is like," he suddenly said aloud. "What a joy."

The idea of looking for positive images of death came among others from the American psychotherapist Stanley Keleman, who proposed this in his book, *Living Your Dying* (1984). But as is expressed in the title, our death is not constrained to the end of life. Every separation contains death on the level of feelings. (Caruso dedicated his book, *The Separation of the Lovers*, to the—emotional—death of his patient at the end of analysis.) F. Perls has most likely supported the spread of "his" "Gestalt"-therapy because the concept of death is so clearly represented in it: "To suffer one's death and to be reborn is not easy," he says. He emphasizes in his book, *Gestalt-Therapy*

Verbatim (1969): The deepened understanding of the "conditio humana" seems to be inevitably joined with the knowledge that the mortal has to be integrated. Goethe (1943) formulated "West oestlicher Diwan": "Die and grow." It appears to be typical for man who thinks in the natural science approach, to consider death as an enemy, and to deny that death does not only represent decay and mischief, but can also bring release (especially in states of severe pain of body or mind). Why this is so, and why it is especially the occidental Christian thinking that has developed in this direction, is difficult to answer and exceeds the frame of this contribution. But let us consider one event that constitutes an essential inhibition for our readiness to die: Alfred Adler, founder of individual psychology, in his book, *Death and Neurosis* (1936), reports about a five-year-old boy who got slapped in the face by his aunt and exclaimed, "How can I continue living now that you have humiliated me so much!" And two pages later he says, "Factual death is also equivalent with the end of striving for successful solution of life problems." The many modes of striving to reduce physical death in his importance are known. Mental death, as it is especially on the neurotic's mind, has no less terrifying power. The same type of statement has been made by the psychoanalyst Eissler in his book, *The Psychology of Death* (Eissler, 1978), in a very concise form, "Better dead than castrated."

This is one of the essential keys to the problem of death, if not the most essential one. There is a very frequent contamination of these two terms: The biological end, and, as Adler names it, our spiritual death; i.e., the feeling of being severely and in a humiliating way constrained in life by some super powerful being. As a consequence, death got to be experienced as a disgracing defeat.

It seems worth striving for a clarification of this contamination in therapeutic work, because this gives an opportunity to the patient to work on the narcissistic offense rather than escaping to illusionary fantasies of eternity. When this is achieved, we might manage to find a way of leaving this world, comparable to what Hermann Hesse expresses with utmost subtlety in *Siddartha* (1953, translated by the author):

Siddartha bowed deeply before departure. "I have known it," he said gently. "You will go to the woods?" "I go to the woods, I go to unity," Vasudeva said emphatically. Emphatically he went away; Siddartha's look followed him. With deep joy, with deep severity he watched the other go, saw his steps full of peace, saw his head full of brightness, saw his figure full of light.

A basic precondition for the encouragement of the incurably ill is the encourager's own stability against discouragement. This in turn requires leaving behind mental polarity, in which life is good and death is our enemy, and entering a dual world.

References

Adler, A. Das Todesproblem in der neurose. *Int. Z. f. Individualpsychologie*, 1936, *14*, 1-6.
Bibeltheologisches Worterbuch: *Heil*. Koln: Styria Verlag.
Biblisch-Historisches Handworterbuch. 2. Band, Heilen. Gottingen: Verlag Vandenhoeck u. Ruprecht.
Caruso, A. I. *Die Trennung der Liebenden*. Frankfurt: Verlag Fischer, 1983.
Dreikurs, R. *Psychologie im Klassenzimmer*. Stuttgart: Verlag Kleet, 1968.
Eissler, K. R. *Der sterbende Patient*. Stuttgart: Verlag Frommann-Holzboog, 1978.
Goethe, J. W. West Oestlicher Diwan; Buch des Saengers, "Seelige Sehnsucht." Leipzeig: Dietrich'sche Verlagsbuchhandlung, 1943.
Hesse, H. *Siddartha*. Frankfurt: Verlag Suhrkamp, 1953.
Hollos, I. Briefe eines entronnenen (Istvan Hollos an Paul Federn, 1946). *Psyche 28*, 266-268, 1974.
Keleman, S. *Living your dying*. New York: Random House Inc., 1974.
Messner, R. *Grenzbereich Todeszone*, Kiepenheuer u. Witsch Koln, 136-139, 1978.

Miller, A. *Du sollst nicht merken.* Frankfurt: Verlag Suhrkamp, 1981.

Perls, F. S. *Gestalt Therapy Verbatim.* Lafayette: Real People Press, 1969.

Tolstoi, L. *Der Tod des Iwan Iljitsch.* Stuttgart: Verlag Reclam, 1981.

8

The Spiritual Dimensions of Working With Families in a Medical Setting

Suzanne R. Engelman

Introduction

Working with families in a medical setting provides the health care team with ample opportunity to witness the diverse influences that impact individual patients under their care. One frequently overlooked dimension of family experience in medical settings is the "spiritual"—both as a family experience before injury, and as a factor that emerges spontaneously in response to illness. It is the purpose of this paper to explore some of the ways in which these spiritual experiences may occur and be utilized in the process of working with patients in a medical setting.

Any discussion about spiritual matters is potentially confusing due to the different ways writers use the term. Clarification of the definition of spirtuality used in this paper will therefore precede further discussion.

Perspectives of spirtuality offered by spokespersons of Transpersonal Psychology provide good working definitions of spirituality for the purposes of this paper. Singer (Note 1) sees the transformation of "ego, from the center of consciousness to an organic part of the larger whole" as an essential ingredient of spiritual experience. Bloomfield (1980) cautions that spirituality is not the same as mysticism and the occult, referring to spiritual experiences as ones that "lead to wholeness and integration, irrespective of religious belief or affiliation" (p. 125). The synthesized meaning of the term spiritual used in this paper refers to experiences which lead one to expanded levels of awareness through a process that shifts one beyond ego boundaries to a larger, more encompassing whole, whether this whole is the collective unconscious, the family, culture or the cosmos. The process by which this shift occurs may include dreams, prayer, second-order learning, dealing with crisis, or working with one's family genogram to evidence the invisible links to earlier generations. These processes will be the focus of this paper, and it is important to distinguish spiritual experiences as used in this text to be *different* from traditional religious practice.

Patients and their families undergoing the shock of physical trauma leading to a spinal cord injury or catastrophic illness such as cancer, are in a state of crisis. At these times when we would expect individuals and their families to retreat and tend to their wounds, could we possibly assume spiritual experiences occur? Observations by this author (Engelman, 1986) and others (Jung, 1972; Firman & Vargiu, 1980) suggest that although spiritual experiences may arise as part of a natural, orderly developmental search for greater meaning in one's life, these experiences may have other emergences that are less harmonious and potentially devastating. Spiritual upheaval may come as a result of a major disruption in the person's life such as terminal illness (Bahnson, 1984), death of a loved one, divorce, or other "violent and destructive interventions of fate" (Jung, 1972, p. 164). Conceptually, a model for thinking about how these spiritual upheavals may occur in patients coping to serious illness is as follows:

Normally, families carry on their lives in a way that is molded to fit the ideals of the particular family in its cultural context. Families have concrete, physical roles that they play out according to unacknowledged family rules, alliances and coping strategies. Considering individual dynamics, this more superficial level of self-definition is what Jung refers to as the "persona level of experience" (Jung, 1972, p. 161). This "persona" level is present in the family dynamic and disguises two less obvious, unconscious levels of influence.

The first unconscious level is the transgenerational family level, which contains the unconscious patterns of behaviors that have been experienced in generations preceding the current family and levels of family awareness that cannot be understood by linear means (Taub-Bynum, 1985). These family patterns are unconsciously passed down and may include specific symptoms, unconscious family myths, roles and the less understandable phenomenon of paranormal family dreams and experiences. The experiences and feeling of a particular family have been repeated over many generations to form an archetypal context that is unconsciously "transmitted" to the current family generation, even though the family member may not have even known his predecessors (Bahnson, Note 2).

The second and deeper unconscious level is what Jung calls the "collective unconscious," or the repository of experiences that underlie all of humanity, including the intensely horrible and beautiful images and feelings that arise during times of spiritual crisis (Jung, 1972, p. 160). Out of this level emerges a living picture, "containing pretty much everything that moves upon the checkerboard of the world, the good and the bad, the fair and the foul" (Jung, 1972, p. 148).

Patients who are undergoing severe disabling and life threatening trauma appear to be catapulted into a crisis situation. Pain, unfamiliarity with strange people and equipment, side effects from strong medication and fear, all accompany the crisis of the immediate illness can lead to a breakdown of the persona level of functioning. This "persona breakdown" may produce a state of disequilibrium that parallels a psychotic disturbance, yet differs from psychosis only from the fact that "dissolution of the persona leads in the end to greater health, while the latter leads only to greater destruction. It is a condition of panic, of letting go in the face of apparently hopeless complications" (Jung, 1972, p. 161).

With the persona somewhat dismantled, forces burst out of

the collective psyche and have a confusing and blinding effect; the plunge into this state may be unavoidable whenever the necessity arises of overcoming an extreme stress in life (Jung, 1972). It is at this time of intense and frequently overwhelming crisis that spiritual dimensions and bizarre behaviors may simultaneously emerge, while patients are being treated in the otherwise rational and organized world of the medical ward. All the metaphors of the larger Self may emerge at this time—God, Jesus, nirvana, prayer, nature, omniscience, and the ultimate truths about life may be revealed with the upsurge of the collective unconscious into conscious awareness. Indeed, as one physician writes of his revelations during an incurable illness,

> My mind is more alive and vivid than ever before...My sensitivities are keener; my affections strong. I seem for the first time to see the world in clear perspective. I love people more deeply and comprehensively. I seem to be just beginning to learn my business and see my work in its proper relationship to science as a whole. I seem to myself to have entered into a period of strong feelings and saner understandings (Cousins, 1983, p. 231).

Thus, while coping to physical illness, the person may experience intensely uplifting or overwhelming feelings of chaos. *How the person copes* may depend on a combination of pre-morbid *personality patterns* and the *kind of support given by the health-care team.* According to Jung (1972), one way in which the person may struggle with the spiritual crisis that ensues is to be overwhelmed by the collective contents, in which case paranoia or schizophrenia may develop. A second way of coping with the upsurge of collective images may be to totally reject them, in which case the person reverts back to an "infantile attitude." This person patches up the persona in order to function in the world, but does so at a level that leaves the full functioning of the person compromised (Jung, 1972, p. 162). The most ideal type of reaction would be that of critical understanding (Jung, 1972). In this mode of coping, the person does not become overly discouraged by the overwhelming images and circumstances, but strives to integrate them, continues to take healthy risks, but with a more cautious understanding that life presents us with challenges that are sometimes beyond our individual control.

As we look into families' backgrounds, we are likely to see the seeds of their religious beliefs that may be contributing to their current coping styles. Patients who are undergoing the shock of serious illness frequently call upon God to relieve their anguish. This pattern may be a reflection of early childhood experiences of religion in which the family called upon God in times of trouble (Singer, 1973).

Seriously ill persons experience their illnesses differently from one another. Many see their illness as just punishment for past sins (Bahnson, Note 2, p. 20), or they may feel that their illness happened as part of a larger pattern in which something is to be learned; that it is God's will. For such persons, belief in a higher power's ultimate plan helps them come to accept their pain and relieve guilt feelings surrounding their past sins (Power & Dell Orto, 1980). Faith in God may also assist those who are overwhelmed with their feelings of hopelessness and powerlessness. Despair has been found to be greatest when a person feels both hopeless and powerless. Being a patient in a medical setting week after week, month after month, is the perfect medium for developing a good case of powerlessness, let alone having a serious illness which further creates physical changes, leaving the person very dependent on others temporarily or permanently. So although the patient may not feel like his or her fate can be controlled (i.e., [s]he feels powerless), one can still come to feel hopeful, by placing what happened to oneself in God's hands. In this way one's faith can be sustaining (Stotland, 1969). This hope, in turn, may facilitate a more optimistic attitude and enhance the healing process.

Bahnson (1984) has also discussed the role of religious experience as it occurs with the terminally ill, as a "denial of nonexistence" which may be

> either helpful or destructive, dependent on whether it constitutes a flight from the solution of urgent interper-

sonal problems, or whether it becomes part of the mosaic of security characterizing the final stage of acceptance of death (p. 250).

Prayer, meditations and visualization are tools that people may use in putting themselves in the kind of psychological space that takes them away from their immediate ego and bodily concerns, and puts them into an altered state of consciousness whereby their awareness may be expanded (Bahnson, Note 2, p. 19). Prayer is frequently used by persons coping with catastrophic illness, and many of the patients with whom I worked have talked about the importance prayer has played for them in their healing process.

Whether or not the prayers hold the conscious desire to obtain something or to have that something "descend" on ourselves or others, the upward projection of feelings has the effect of "lifting" the center of consciousness in some measure into subtler levels of the inner world. It is a process of elevating feelings, and desires, and thus transmuting them into aspirations toward higher goals (Firman et al., 1980, p. 111).

This paper will now focus upon three specific instances of patients integrating spiritual experiences as part of coping to their serious illness. The genogram, which is a diagram of the family's three generational structure, is used to facilitate the patient and family's recognition of the role of transgenerational problems and the role of spirituality in the past. These genograms are included with each case presentation.

The first case is that of Joe, a 23 year old man who sustained a spinal cord injury during a hang-gliding accident two years ago. I worked with him during his initial hospitalization and had the opportunity to meet with him again during a subsequent hospitalization for diagnosis of abdominal pain. Joe represents the struggle of many spinal cord injured persons; most, however, do not have outcomes as positive as Joe's. Prayer was a very important aspect of Joe's rehabilitation. Like many spinal cord injured patients, he asked and was told within a few days of his accident, that he would "never walk again." At that time, paralyzed from the shoulders down, Joe responded that that was unacceptable to him and he would walk out of the rehab center. The medical staff felt he was "in denial," because they had diagnosed him as a C-4 Quadraplegic, Frankel Class A, with a one out of one hundred chances of ever walking. Later he was told his chances of walking were more like one in one thousand.

Like many spinal cord injured patients, Joe prayed a lot— 24 hours a day. Joe also thought a lot about his father who at

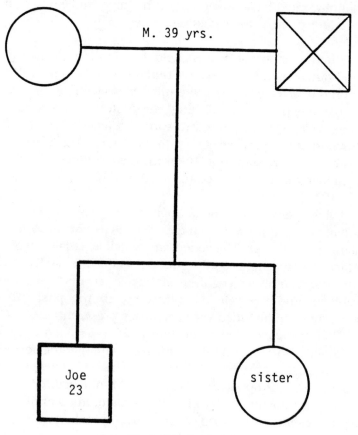

Illustration #1: Joe

one time developed cancer and was bedridden for many years, but eventually "overcame it—I knew that if he could do it, I could too. So I spent a lot of time praying and thinking about how he did it." Especially during the first six weeks of his rehabilitation, before any part of Joe's body began to move, his feelings needed particular uplifting; but after he started getting movement back in his hands, then his toes, the physical proof was uplifting enough.

Joe did "walk out" of the hospital to return home to live with his father and work on strengthening himself so he could walk more functionally. Most patients do not leave the hospital with as good an outcome, but then again, maybe most patients did not have the same inner experiences about overcoming illness and conviction that Joe had. Joe's own feelings were that his prayers and the optimism they engendered were what got him walking.

The second case study regards Jarl, a 50 year old man, who came from a "long line of healers" in his family. His great-grandmother who lived in the Mid-West, used to do natural healing with herbs and laying on of hands. She was a full Cherokee Indian and passed her healing down to her children, which Jarl was very comfortable talking to me about but indicated, "It's the kind of stuff I wouldn't tell just anybody, and certainly not the doctors. They would think I'm 'nuts.'" Jarl talked about the time his great-grandmother walked several miles through the woods to tell her daughter that something was wrong with the oldest male child of her string of nine children. At that time John was fine, only to come down with polio two days after the grandmother's prophecy. In his own generation, Jarl talked about his mother's psychic abilities to know when her children were in trouble. She "had a feelin' about this accident when it happened," just as Jarl too, had had a feeling of expectation before he had his vehicle accident. "All along I had been saying to myself that I shouldn't be going." When he got to the underpass that people had warned him about before he left that day, he was "struck by a blinding wall of white light" and never knew what hit him.

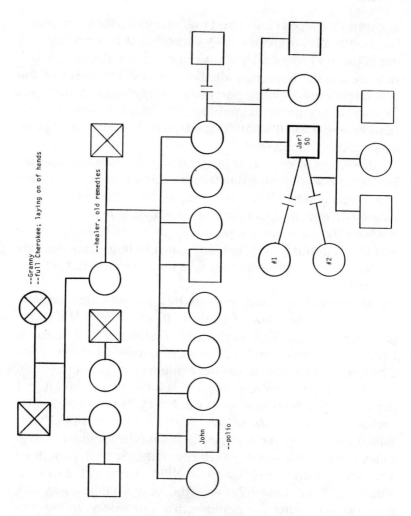

Illustration #2: Jarl

For the first several weeks after his accident, Jarl fought for his life. His injury had been so debilitating that his lungs stopped working on their own. He had to use a respirator, which breathed for him. Three times his breathing stopped while he was on the respirator. One of those times was due to the respirator malfunctioning. Because of his past history with "spiritual" experiences, Jarl had the inner resources to help him cope with the severe panic and terror of losing his breath and suffocating. Jarl talked about how he was able to teach himself to breath again by

> focusing on the square I put in my lungs. When I focused on the square, it would gradually get larger and it was white light. Gradually it expanded until it filled my whole lungs and then I could breath totally on my own. If my concentration was interrupted just the slightest, the square would disappear and I would have to start over again. On the other hand, I couldn't really fully focus on the square because that could interfere too.

Unknown to him at that time, Jarl had described the process of meditation and passive volition in the act of focusing. Jarl was busy in his process of "inspiring" himself. As the psychologist working with Jarl, I gave him much support to continue along the path he was on and praised him for the excellent way in which he worked with his own inner healer.

Finally, I would like to end with the story of Janice, who was a 48 year old woman with metastatic breast cancer. Janice opened her life to me about nine months before she was to die. Her goals were to be able to have help in looking at and going through the process which she felt would end in death.

Janice had been the sixth born of eight girls in the rural farm country of North Dakota. Life was hard on the farm, and her father, disappointed in not having any sons, expected his daughters to see to the farm work. By the time chores were done, Janice didn't have much time for social life. When she was 32, she met her future husband and they were soon married. While she was pregnant with their son, Dave, her husband developed multiple sclerosis. By the time her baby was delivered, her husband was going into a wheelchair. He gradually deteriorated and when Dave was 8 years old, his father died. Janice was 39 and completely in charge of bringing up her young son and her deceased husband's two teenage daughters from a previous marriage. Nine years later, Janice was diagnosed with metastatic breast cancer.

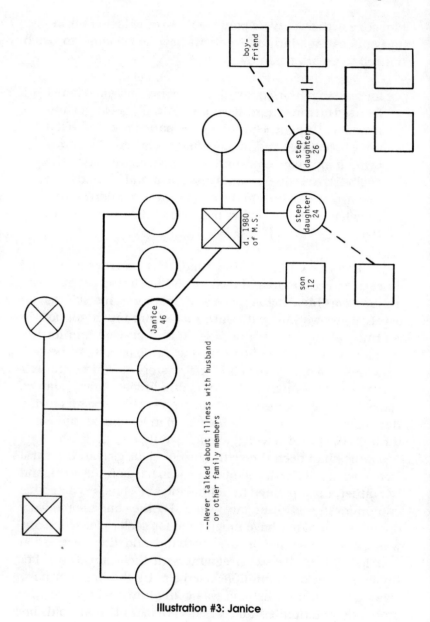

Illustration #3: Janice

As we talked about these early life events, Janice explored regrets she had. One of the major issues for her was that she had never been able to talk to her husband or any other family members in the process of his dying. Her fears were that her death would be an equally lonely experience. Janice wanted to do it differently. As hard as it would be, she wanted to bring family tensions, cut-offs, and other feelings out into the open. In particular, she wanted to know her son better, and role model the process of communicating for him. She was concerned about Dave's very quiet and sometimes moody nature.

This precipitated the beginnings of family meetings. Throughout the course of the next nine months, we had many family sessions; at the times when Janice would deteriorate physically and her sisters would fly in from other parts of the country, they would be included. Janice was anxious to try anything that would help to alleviate her anguish in facing her impending death. We used hypnosis to help with the periodic headaches and pain; visualizations to "chart" the growth of her cancer at times when the physicians were unable to clinically diagnose its spread; and just honest heart to heart discussions among all the family members. Janice experienced all of these events as enlarging upon the quality of her life, while struggling with tremendous resistance to stay open to herself and her family.

Previously closed to expressions of anger, Janice was able to really let her anger out about her progressing sickness. As she began to make her transition into another reality closer to death, Janice bitterly cried, "I can't believe this is happening to me." She vented her frustration with her family's difficulties dealing with her loss of memory and disorientation, but during her final days, Janice had to be reminded that her mind and body were turning inward and she need not be judgmental of her failing cognitive abilities and hair loss. In other words, I worked with Janice to release some of her ego concerns to look and act appropriately and prepare for a larger reality.

Her resistance to death continued up until the final day. A hospital bed was set up in her bedroom. She tossed and turned in her bed, bolting upright with her small frail hands grabbing the rail of her bed, only to fall back again, gently into her depths. And finally came the day of Janice's death. Within an hour of her death, I arrived at her home and together with family members, including her three children, two sisters and two friends, we encircled her bed. Taking Janice's hands, we kneeled around her bed and formed an energy circle to say our good-byes and talk about what we had loved about Janice, and had been troubled by. It was a tremendously powerful time for us all, leaving our everyday world to spend these last few moments in the sanctuary of Janice's room, as she speeded off into another realm. Each person said their good-byes in their own special ways. Our circle included Janice and respected her dying wishes. Just as we had met as a family together throughout the process of her dying, so we completed the process with Janice.

These three case presentations underscore the importance of considering the whole family system within which the patient is embedded. The current family and previous generations may all affect how the patient deals with serious illness. Spiritual experiences (as opposed to traditional religious practice) have been overlooked as an important ingredient in dealing with illness, and need to be respected as part of the whole experience of coping to serious illness.

Reference Notes

1. Singer, J. Personal communication, Palo Alto, CA, August 13, 1986.
2. Bahnson, C. B. Disability in classical myth and modern society. Presented at a workshop/seminar at the Woodrow Wilson International Center for Scholars, Smithsonian Institute, Washington, D.C., May 13, 1981.

References

Bahnson, C. B. Psychosomatic issues in cancer. In R. L. Gallon (Ed.), *The psychosomatic approach to illness.* New York: Elsevier-North Holland, 1983.

Bahnson, C. B. Psychological aspects of cancer. In Y. H. Pilch (Ed.), *Surgical oncology.* New York: McGraw-Hill Book Co., 1984.

Bloomfield, H. Transcendental meditation as an adjunct to therapy. In S. Boorstein (Ed.), *Transpersonal psychotherapy*. Palo Alto, CA.: Science and Behavior, 1980.

Cousins, N. *The healing heart*. New York: W. W. Norton, 1983.

Engelman, S. R. Clinical approaches to care of the terminally ill family. *International Journal of Psychosomatics*, 1986, *33(2)*, 48-50.

Firman, J., & Vargiu, J. Personal and transpersonal growth: the perspective of psychosynthesis. In S. Boorstein (Ed.), *Transpersonal psychotherapy*. Palo Alto, CA.: Science and Behavior Books, 1980.

Jung, C. G. *Two essays on analytical psychology*. Princeton, N.J.: Bollingen Series XX, 1972.

Power, P., & Dell Orto, A. Impact of disability/illness on the adult. In P. Power and A. E. Dell Orto (Eds.), *Role of the family in the rehabilitation of the physically disabled*. Texas: ProEd, 1980.

Singer, J. Jung as a spiritual teacher. *Revision Magazine*, 1985, *4*, 10-18.

Stotland, E. *The psychology of hope*. New York: Josey-Bass, 1969.

Taub-Bynum, E. *The family unconscious: the enfolding field*. New York: Quest, 1985.

9

The Family's Roles in Health and Disease

Stephen Fleck

Family physicians and family medicine have been with us for a long time. Traditionally "the doctor's job" meant to know and tend to all members in a family, bringing them to life and attending them while dying. Without having been taught what this group of people is about, how to understand what they are supposed to be doing as a unit or how they might be deficient as a family, he could intuitively sense that some of them functioned or behaved more effectively than others. He might even have suspected now or then that a family's ailments or problems might be generated from within it. Of course, there was little occasion to consider such matters for any length of time because most illnesses to be attended to were acute pneumonias in the winter and intestinal infections in the summer with epidemics of severe child infections interspersed. Only since the major infectious illnesses have been prevented or rendered treatable and modern surgery mastered how to deal with serious trauma or tumors, has it become apparent that the so-called chronic and degenerative diseases including major mental illnesses are certainly influenced and possibly engendered in part by psychosocial factors.

Psychosomatic concepts had arisen early in this century, beginning with Weizsäcker in Germany and through the work of Pavlov and Cannon who influenced clinicians like Carl Binger, Flanders Dunbar, and Felix Deutsch who in turn had a firsthand view of Sigmund Freud's psychosomatic frailties (Cannon, 1929; Binger, Ackerman, Cohn, Schoeder & Steele, 1945; Dunbar, 1976; Deutsch & Murphy, 1967). But they and others sought specific personality features related to particular conditions like hypertension or peptic ulcer (Dunbar, 1976; Alexander, 1948). In line with Freud who eschewed consideration of family pathology (Freud, 1941) and limited his clinical focus to the intrapsychic, the specificity research focussed on psychosomatic issues in the narrow sense of that concept.

Only toward the middle of this century was research concerning social factors begun, but not of families as a relevant factor (Mirsky, 1958; Hinkle & Wolf, 1952). Yet, one pioneering study by Richardson summarized in a Monograph, *Patients Have Families* (Richardson, 1948) was largely ignored, although he described in great detail and clarity the cybernetic interactions between patients and their families as an important co-variant in the course of an illness. In general, over the past thirty years we have witnessed a tremendous increment in clinical and scientific interest in the family and in family treatment in particular, although studies of families' roles in illness have been relatively few. One outstanding work has recently been published in the U.S.: Huygen's *Family Medicine*, an insightful account of family practice over several decades (Huygen, 1982).

There are two major facets to the family's role in medicine to be considered. One is the family as a possible source or contributor to illness, and the other concerns the family's caretaker mission in health and illness. As to the first facet aside from genetic factors, it is less than 50 years since some pioneers began to wonder about and investigate the unusual family frame in which obese and some diabetic children lived, and others noted the very strange family backgrounds of schizophrenic patients (Bruch, 1940; Lidz & Lidz, 1949; Midelfort, 1957).Documentation of family pathology in the background of young schizophrenic patients (Lidz, Fleck & Cornelison, 1965; Lidz & Lidz, 1949) and the development of family therapy in lieu of or in addition to the treatment of children (Ackerman & Behrens, 1977) led psychiatrists and many more other mental health professionals to exploit these findings therapeutically. But concerns with delineating normative or wholesome family functioning let alone establishing typologies has remained sparse. It is claimed by many, but seriously apprehended by few, that the most useful procedure in understanding and conceptualizing the family as an institution is a general systems approach, allowing for ordering the multi-faceted relationships and constant changes in this system (Bertalanffy, 1968).

Also we hear today a great deal about the decline or deterioration of the family as have most generations before us since ancient times, but it is obvious that an institution that has existed and survived for thousands of years is not going to disappear, but necessarily will change, much as we would not consider Greek democracy a democratic way for us to live by today. Within the framework of a general system which can be defined as a collectivity of specifiable elements in particular relationships which interact in cybernetic fashion, the family is but one system or sub-system in a hierarchy which ranges from cells to the universe. In this hierarchy the family is interposed between every individual and the family's community (see Table 1).

Table 1
A Hierarchy of Living Matter

Viruses	mostly sub-microscopic; live matter composed of nucleic acids (the key substance for inheritance) and proteins or protein building stones.
Cells	complex units with nuclei and various constituents, e.g., mitochondria, membranes (boundaries), tails for locomotion, etc.
Organs	consist of connected and communicating cells of s single cell type or limited number of different types cells.

Organisms	any composite of organs permitting independent existence as a unit (unlike organs, but like bacteria, i.e., single cells). Propagation usually depends on contributions from two organisms through gametes (male and female) among plants and animals.
Group and Family	aggregation of like species organisms; in higher animals survival depends on bi-generational social arrangements. In the human race biologically related families may form larger kinships across several generations and distant collaterals.
Community	consists of biologically unrelated families and individuals who share living space and fulfill complementary roles, helping each other, freeing up energy for non-subsistence activities.
Nations	collection of communities which join for mutual advantages, protection or acquisitive pursuits.
World	the total of our planet with all living and inanimate constituents.
Solar System	collection of planets and satellites gyrating around the sun, the basic source of life as we know it, which does not exist on other planets.
Universe	the space surrounding the solar system with other solar systems and stars and structures barely perceived or understood by us.

The family may constitute a system complex spanning several generations and collaterals, and these forms vary among societies and over time. Minimally the family must be defined as a two-generational system, no matter how many or few persons in each generation. Furthermore, it usually consists of members of two generations who are biologically related, the older generation having produced the younger one, although family status can be accorded by law or similar societal rules. In general, the family has three missions: to procreate; to protect and nurture the young; and to prepare the young for membership as adults in their communities, however adulthood may be defined. Clearly the first two missions are life preserving for the race and for the young respectively; enculturation, the third mission may or may not be left to the family or the parents as such. In some societies sons are removed from their parents or their mothers if the parents do not live together, and brought up in special programs where boys are to become or to be made into men.

In Western society for the most part all three missions are left to the primary family group or to the extended family, but increasingly to the bi-generational nuclear family when societies have moved toward industrialization and modernization of life.

Industrialization and mobility led to a degree of isolation of the nuclear family which has rendered the personalities of the parents and their coalition more critical as the sole leaders and models for children in representing relationship modes, gender identity and role examples. This relative isolation has also accentuated the basic triangular structure of the family group with two parents as leaders and children as followers which must be appreciated. Each child lives in a different triangle in addition to sibling relationships, which only the firstborn will not have for a period of time.

Turning from historical glimpses to the clinical examination of the family, we propose a five-pronged systems view of the family (Fleck, 1983).

The five foci for the examination of human systems are: Leadership, Boundaries, Affectivity, Communication, and Task and Goal Performance. These parameters, their relationship with personality development and structure and their sub-division for clinical scrutiny are presented in Figure 1 and Table 2. This scheme provides for historical and cross-sectional assessments.

The Family's Roles in Health and Disease

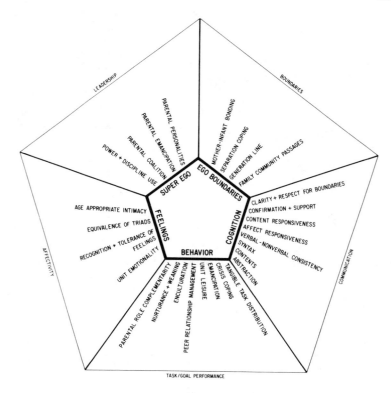

Figure 1. Foci of Human Systems

Leadership is vested in the marital pair, and as already indicated, their relationship as well as their respective personalities are critical in guiding the family through its life cycle, which begins with pregnancy and birth and ends, in one sense, with the emancipation of the young into adult society.

Boundaries are essential in any system; they define the system and sub-systems or organization and need to be managed or controlled with regard to exchanges across a boundary. In the case of the family, three boundaries matter: (a) the rather intangible ego boundaries which children must acquire during their development; (b) the generation boundary which divides the adults and leaders from the younger generation who must grow and learn and also represents the incest

Table 2
5 Foci of Human Systems

Leadership	Boundaries	Affectivity	Communication	Task/Goal Performance
Parental personalities	Parental sub-system. Ego boundary development in children	Inter-parental intimacy	Clarity as to forum, syntax and contents	Nurturance and weaning
Marital coalition	Generation boundary	Equivalence of family cathexes in triads	Affect-responsiveness. Contents-responsiveness	Separation mastery (toddling)
Parental role complementarities	Age-appropriate family community permeability	Tolerance for feelings and their expression	Verbal/nonverbal consistency	Behavior control and guidance and oedipal passage
Use of power and discipline		Unit emotionality (celebrations and mourning)	Expressivity	Peer relationship management
			Abstract thinking	Unit activities and leisure
				Crisis coping
				Emancipation
				Post-nuclear

taboo and (c) the family community-boundary which is rather tangible, and in the case of the family can be managed in terms of time and space.

Affectivity is the cement that holds the family together, especially so in modern urban societies where there is often only one breadwinner and children are no asset or advantage in procuring the group's basic living needs. An atmosphere of love and caring is essential for the optimal growth and development of all family members. The related exercise of power and discipline in promoting or subverting an atmosphere of caring in the family is more critical now than in the past, because the sense of familyness in free and developed societies depends on mutual good feeling and no longer on economic necessity or rigid moral codes conduct.

Communication, especially the exchange of information, is fundamental in any system and in the family is a very important learning area for the children. Language and in general the cultural symbols used in the larger community need to be first learned in the family, specifically so in modern societies, for the children's school readiness and their ultimate capacity for formal or abstract operations as defined by Piaget (Bertalanffy, 1968).

The *tasks and goals* of the family begin with the establishment of a marital coalition and then consist of the creation of a new generation, their nurturance, enculturation and their graduation into adult society. Thus, the family as a unit must be guided through many different life stages related to the individual development of family members, and eventually the parents must face as a pair non-parental roles, grandparenthood and eventually decline and death. Strictly speaking the family life cycle comes to closure sometime during parental midlife or somewhat later, but also continues by overlapping with the new family life cycles created by "children." When old age supervenes, children may have to assume quasi-parental leadership responsibilities for aging and possibly handicapped parents, especially now when longevity is much more common.

Besides coping with the various life cycle transitions, often entailing painful separation mastery like school entry of a child, the family also must manage unforeseeable crises like illness, economic reverses, etc., and it may be reiterated that among all "health care providers" the family ranks first in both acute and chronic illness care.

Among family tasks the role in health education needs to be emphasized. Habits concerning eating, exercise, personal hygiene and other health measures are formed and learned early in life, usually under the aegis of the family; specifically the parents' examples to be followed. Parental dietary habits as well as their foibles with regard to substance abuse, their coping with anxieties—all these are copied or absorbed by children, sometimes negatively so, because older children may decide to do the opposite of what their parents indulged in or abstained from.

One of the earliest family studies was conducted by Hilde Bruch (Bruch, 1940) and concerned the unusual "family frame" of diabetic and obese children. This was at a time when the emphasis and search for specificity in psychosomatic conditions was in the ascendency, tying illnesses like asthma or ulcerative colitis to particular personality constellations, although many clinicians had observed that the mothers of colitis patients usually were over-involved with such children. Familial pathology in medical conditions cannot be presented here in detail except to indicate that in our assessment scheme it is often close to that of psychotic patients in a family as indicated in Table 3.

In addition to our systems assessment scheme, the genogram provides an important overview of families, as well as an opportunity to work with a family in establishing their own history and situation. Its usefulness will be illustrated together with a couple of clinical vignettes (Fig. 2 and Fig. 3).

The first (Fig. 2) is that of a young woman who developed fulminating ulcerative colitis while on a trip to Mexico with her husband to whom she had been married less than two years. He began an affair with a friend of the patient's who accompanied them. Developing diarrhea in Mexico does not make one think quickly of a serious illness, but this young woman became seriously ill quickly and perforated within a few weeks

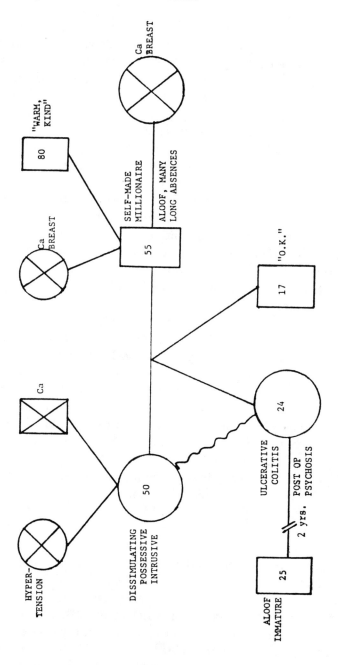

Figure 2. Ulcerative Colitis

just prior to scheduled surgery. Her past medical and psychiatric history were unremarkable, but following the operation she became acutely psychotic, tried to strangle her mother who had come to help nurse her and refused all nourishment and eventually had to be transferred to a psychiatric ward despite satisfactory surgical healing per se and a well-functioning ileostomy. She literally fought against eating.

Her parents had been married nearly thirty years, although lived separately much of the time as the father, a self-made businessman did a great deal of traveling and maintained an apartment in a distant city. He had very little to do with his daughter's upbringing, therefore, and on the whole they had a bland unemotional relationship. During her illness, however, he took command, flew in consultants from other cities, but disappeared after the operation before the patient was even conscious after the surgeon had advised him that she was out of acute danger.

The mother had been a teacher for a few years prior to her marriage, but became a full-time housewife after her marriage, overattending to her daughter for as long as she stayed at home. This overattending consisted of close attention to every move and function of the daughter's, including her bodily functions all through high school, monitoring her dates and being involved in the daughter's extra-curricular activities such as dancing and art lessons to which the mother always transported her daughter and waited until the end of the lesson to take her home. When this girl went to college a short distance from home she felt quite disoriented at first, but quickly adjusted without professional help, made friends, promptly fell in and out of love a number of times and in her senior year became engaged and married. The marriage proved difficult; except for sexual satisfaction there was little they shared or found interesting in each other and the trip to Mexico actually was an attempt to shore up their marriage or at least make it more meaningful. When the patient became sick, however, and especially when the husband learned about the necessity of a colostomy he immediately distanced himself, visited very little and very briefly, and after her transfer to the psychiatric ward remained absent except for one interview with a social worker. He was not only unable to accept her physical impairment, but also was uninterested in trying to make any accomodation to her misfortune. They were divorced before the patient had recovered.

The patient's younger and only sibling, a brother, was then in high school and according to the parents doing very well, but according to the sister was an "unhappy, isolated kid."

The patient gradually improved and became involved in intensive psychotherapy over a number of years, eventually remarried, became an artist, and has remained well.

The family as a system was deficient in practically all parameters. Leadership was impaired in that the mother was intrusive, almost as if trying to lead her daughter's life, the father physically absent a great deal and emotionally absent all the time. There was no real coalition between the parents and very little communication.

Boundaries were deficient because of the mother's intrusiveness which violated both the patient's sense of ego and the generation boundary. It is possible, or at least the patient suspected later on that her mother might have had homosexual feelings toward her. The family's life was constricted in that the patient was not helped to develop peer relationships while living at home, although she had little trouble entering into sexual relationships without appreciating that other dimensions were lacking in these encounters which she did not realize until after she was married for some time.

Family affectivity was deficient in that the father was distant and seemingly cold, the mother over-involved, but not attentive to her children's feelings and emotional growth needs.

Communication was relatively intact, at least cognitively, although the mother spoke for the daughter in many ways, as already indicated, and the father eventually turned out to be a very unreliable, not to say dishonest, informant. He kept many secrets with regard to his activities and business, although there is no evidence that he had affairs or significant liaisons outside the marriage. However, language about feelings was

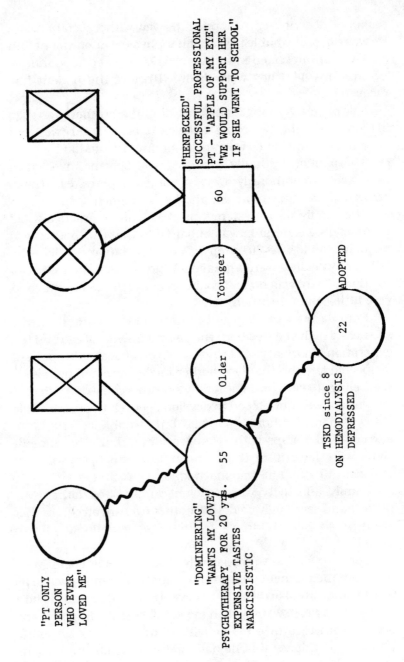

Figure 3. Hemodialysis

practically non-existent, and the patient literally had to learn a good deal in this respect in therapy.

Family tasks with regard to development were outwardly fulfilled, except there was never any stage of real family cohesion, although they were usually together on holidays. A tentative assessment score for this family was 3.3 close to the range of families with a psychotic member.

The second illustration is of a 22 year old, single, unemployed young woman, a college drop-out on hemodialysis for twelve years who was referred because of psychotic depression with more self-destructive behavior than suicidal preoccupation (Figure 3). She was aware, however, of the dangers of her indulgence in alcohol and marijuana, and her neglect of dietary restrictions, especially with regard to potassium-containing foods and drinks. She dreamt she might be God and was afraid "to lose my mind."

She had been adopted shortly after delivery by an Ivy-league graduate student according to what she was told by her parents who emphasized for as long as she can remember that she had been "chosen."

Outwardly her development and family life were without trouble until at age eight she developed focal nephritis secondary to an antibiotic administered for a streptococcal infection. Her kidneys failed to recover and she entered TSKD within a year. There followed a number of trips to a medical center 300 miles away involving assessments, dialysis and two cadaver transplants, the first being rejected over four years and the second within one year. The patient has remained on hemodialysis since 1976. She continued her schooling, however, throughout and lost only one year, graduating with honors and getting into the college of her parents' choice. She had no real interest in a college career and wanted to pursue her musical interests, reputedly based on considerable talent, and quit college after three semesters.

Her parents, married for 30 years, considered themselves happy, their only problem and disappointment allegedly being their daughter's failure to continue with and graduate from college. They also objected to her lifestyle and refused any joint sessions with the daughter. However, the mother has been in personal psychotherapy for more than 20 years and according to the patient the mother runs the family and the father is afraid to oppose her (which I could confirm through phone contacts, and which had previously been noted in family interviews by a colleague). The parents feel that the patient has treated them badly and it is difficult to get the mother off the theme, "after all that I have been through with my daughter's illness, she does this to me," i.e., dropping out of school. Although very affluent they have refused to support the patient despite her repeated need for hospital care for cardiac arrest, uterine and G.I. bleeding.

From a systems standpoint we are dealing with skewed parental leadership where the mother's narcissistic needs take precedence over family needs. This leadership defect became overt only with the patient's unfortunate medical condition.

Boundaries are generally intact, although the patient has some difficulties in maintaining ego boundaries in intimate relationships.

Affectivity is distorted, love conditional on carrying out parental goals and the patient is denied love when pursuing independent goals. This rigid emphasis on adhering to mother's needs and definition for success is a common seedbed for later depression, which brought the patient to psychiatric treatment. It is also one of the crassest instances of pathological delegation as defined by Stierlin (Fleck, 1983).

Communication seemed adequate or better except for the content around the patient's independence strivings.

Task performance also seemed effective until the emancipation stage, as described. The mother and the father to a lesser degree cared for the patient through the period of her chronic illness and disablement, but withdrew from the task when the patient pursued her emancipation from them, seeking her independence. The tentative assessment score in this case was 2.75, a mid-range family.

Both cases illustrate significant contributions of family pathology to the course of illness, and in the first example a possible etiological role as well. Typical assessment findings according to our scheme are illustrated in Table 3 showing psycho-physiologic disorders in the high, but not highest range of family pathology.

In summary, I have attempted to present an overview of the general role and missions of the family in human life and some specifics about familial factors in health and disease. The two aspects—the family as health care provider, a task in which both families presented here failed, and the family as an etiological contributor to illness, a likelihood in the first case illustrated.

Clinical assessment of family competence applicable in medical practice has been presented utilizing the Yale Guide to Family Assessment and genograms. The assessment is based on a five-pronged systems analyses estimating respectively the qualities of leadership, boundary management, affectivity, communication and task and goal performance through the life cycle. These evaluations are based on the premise of what most families accomplish individually at various stages to safeguard and promote wholesome development and existence.

The genogram, a quick overview of family structure over at least three generations, highlights the clinically relevant relationships and conditions, as illustrated with two examples.

It needs to be emphasized that human health, the wholesome balance between an organism and its inanimate and animate environment, is contingent on family competence as a system. In illness we need to consider not only psychosomatic and somato-psychic mechanisms, but also familio-somatic and somato-familial factors as presented so cogently over the years by Claus Bahne Bahnson (Bahnson, 1983).

Table 3
Family Scores Typical For Four Disorders

Schizophrenia: X   Affective Disorder: O   Psychophysiological Disorders: *
Neurotic Disorder: +   No diagnosed disorder: −

Rating Scale		0 (Not rated)	1 (Adequate or better)	2 (Somewhat deficient)	3 (Moderately deficient)	4 (Aberrant)	5 (Grossly aberrant)
Parameter: Leadership	Parental personalities		−	+	O	*	X
	Parents' emancipation	O +	−			*X	
	Mutual support	+ −			O	*	X
	Power use			−	+	O*	X
Boundary Management	Mother-child dyad	−		+ O		*	X
	Separation coping	+ −			*	O	X
	Generation boundary	O −		+ *			X
	Family-community passages			− *	O +		X
Affectivity	Age-appropriate intimacy	−		O +	*		X
	Equivalence of triads	+ O		− +		X	
	Tolerance for feelings		−		+ O*	X	
	Unit emotionality	−		+ *	O		X
Communication	Clarity and respect for boundaries	O + −				*	X
	Confirmation and support		−	O	+ *		X
	Content responsiveness		− +	O *			X
	Affect responsiveness			− +	O	*	X
	Verbal/nonverbal consistencies		+ −		O *		X
	Syntax	− O + *			X		
	Contents	− O +		*			X
	Abstraction	− O +					X
Task Fulfillment	Parental-role complementarity	+ O −				*	X
	Nurturance and weaning			−	+	*	O X
	Enculturation		−	*	O +	X	
	Peer-relationship management		−	+ *	O X		
	Unit leisure			− * + O			X
	Emancipation		−	* + O			X
	Crisis coping	− + O		*	X		
	Tangible tasks and distribution	+		− *	X O		

Scores (Total divided by 28):   No Diag. 1.4; Neurotic 1.8; Affective 2.3; Psychophysiol. 2.7; Schizophrenic 4.5

References

Ackerman, N. W., & Behrens, M. L. Family diagnosis and clinical process. In G. Caplan (Ed.), *American handbook of psychiatry* (Vol. 2), 1977.

Alexander, F. *Fundamentals of psychoanalysis*. New York: W. W. Norton, 1948.

Bahnson, C. B. Individual and family response to external and internal stress, Proceedings of the Seventh World Congress of Psychiatry, Vienna, 1983, in press.

Bateson, G., Jackson, D., Haley, J., & Weakland, H. Toward a theory of schizophrenia. *Behavioral Science*, 1956, *1*, 251-264.

Bertalanffy, L. von. *Organismic psychology and systems theory*. Worcester: Clark University Press, 1968.

Binger, C. A., Ackerman, N. W., Cohn, A. F., Schoeder, H. A., & Steele, J. H. Personality in arterial hypertension, *Psychosomatic Medicine Monographs*. New York: Hoeber, 1945.

Bruch, H. The family frame of obese children. *Psychosomatic Medicine*, 1940, *2*, 141-206.

Cannon, W. B. *Bodily changes in pain, hunger, fear and rage*. New York: Appleton-Century-Crofts, 1929.

Deutsch, F., & Murphy, W. The Clinical Interview (Vol. 1). Diagnosis: *A method of teaching associative exploration.* (Vol. 2). Therapy: *a method of teaching sector psychotherapy*. New York: International Universities Press, 1967.

Dunbar, H. F. *Emotions and bodily changes: a survey of literature on psychosomatic interrelationships 1910-1953* (4th ed.). New York: Ayer Company, 1976.

Fleck, S. Evaluation of the family in general medical care. In H. Leigh (Ed.), *Psychiatry in the practice of medicine*. California: Addison-Wesley, 1983.

Freud, S. Eine Probe Psychoanalytischer Arbeit, Gesammelte Werke 17. London: Imago Publishing Company, Ltd., 1941.

Hinkle, L. E., & Wolf, S. A summary of experimental evidence relating life stress to diabetes mellitus. *Journal of Mt. Sinai Hospital*, 1952, *19*, 537.

Huygen, F. J. *Family medicine: the medical life histories of families.* New York: Brunner/Mazel, 1982.

Lidz, R. W., & Lidz, T. The family environment of schizophrenic patients. *American Journal of Psychiatry,* 1949, *106,* 332-345.

Lidz, T., Fleck, S., & Cornelison, A. *Schizophrenia and the family.* New York: International Universities Press, 1965.

Midelfort, C. F. *The family in psychotherapy.* New York: McGraw-Hill, 1957.

Mirsky, I. A. Physiologic, psychologic, and social determinants in etiology of duodenal ulcer. *American Journal Digest,* 1958, *3,* 285.

Richardson, H. B. *Patients have families.* New York: Commonwealth Fund, 1948.

10

On the Threshold of Death: Implications of Impending Death on Patients, Physicians and Families

Dan G. Hertz

Introduction

Statistically, the number of deaths equals exactly the number of births. But whereas the life of any organism is subject to chance and circumstance, its death is an absolute fact. Death is the one thing in life which is entirely certain, but because it can be known only from one side, so to speak, it remains a mystery to man. This difficulty is reflected in our approach to a definition of death. It is defined as a lack of life, but as there exists no good understanding of what life is, no great conceptual advances are gained by such a definition.

Scientists can point to conditions which are necessary for life to occur and likewise, for death, but the status of any of these conditions is not clearly understood. Recent advances in medicine, for example, have questioned the feasibility of using heart-death as a criterion for the end of life, suggesting instead that brain-death is a more appropriate criterion. Whatever the outcome of this and future debates about how to determine the moment of death, death will, in all likelihood, remain a mystery, forever leaving medicine only with increased powers to postpone it, but no closer to preventing it.

Parallel with the considerable advances made by the biological sciences in the study of fatal diseases, psychiatrists have become increasingly involved in studying how the individual faces death. A number of conceptual breakthroughs in how death is viewed may be partly responsible for the growing interest in this area. To describe the background against which these changes have occurred would involve a lengthy review of various views of death which have evolved through the intellectual, religious and spiritual history of man. It is sufficient to say that the more traditional views saw death as a sudden end to life, life otherwise being related in no way to death. In contrast to this, modern views see life and death as intimately related. Regarding death as central to living itself is a cornerstone of the psychoanalytic theories of Freud, the philosophy of Heidegger, and the view of the biologist, Ehrenberg. A natural implication of this approach to death is the emergence of death as a subject of study for analysts and psychiatrists alike.

Three additional factors account for increased efforts to understand how the individual handles death. First, how death is perceived depends upon how life is perceived. Scientific developments as well as functional changes in many modern societies have bestowed upon their individual members unprecedented benefits in terms of comfort and security. In the twentieth century, Western countries are so advanced and sophisticated that the well-being of the individual is a subject which can be pragmatically addressed and, for most purposes, adequately solved. Modern medicine and organization have made it possible to expend considerable efforts to protect the quality of life of the individual. The obvious improvements in the quality of life, however, stand in stark contrast to increased and undisguised manifestations of aggression and violence by which the twentieth century is also characterized.

The growing interest in how the individual faces death may derive from this odd coexistence of the well-demonstrated creative powers of the modern world along with the equally well-demonstrated tendency to destruction.

A second and more specific factor is the impact of the

psychoanalytic school of thought on understanding the individual as a whole. The psychoanalytic view emphasizes the "Why" and "How" of human actions and reactions rather than the more traditional search for an adequate description of the "What" of human activity. This view also enables a comprehensive approach to the psychological study of death.

Last, the importance of developmental and integrational group processes in the family structure, as revealed through therapeutic interaction, has been recognized. This has made possible an assessment of interaction between a dying person and his family as well as an evaluation of the impact of this trying emotional experience on both family members and physicians. The increasing amount of work with families has yielded much information on how death is dealt with. This essay intends to point to and discuss some of the pertinent aspects of this process.

Selected Review of the Literature

Modern psychiatric and psychoanalytic literature set the beginning of modern thanathology at Freud's two essays, "The Theme of the Three Caskets" (1913) and "Thought for the Times on War and Death" (1915). In the first essay, Freud suggested that love may be viewed as a reaction formation to death. In the second, he noted that war between modern countries expresses an underlying aspect of man's nature as a killer, which is more fundamental than man's civilized behavior in times of peace. In this paper Freud also distinguished between the death of an enemy, the death of a loved one and one's own death. Each of these situations has its own dynamics and implications. The death of an enemy is perceived with no afterthought of threat to the individual himself. The death of a loved one, however, sets in motion a number of psychological processes. Although love-hate ambivalence towards a loved one may introduce an element of gratification upon his death, Freud maintained that a part of an individual's ego dies along with the beloved.

Examining the problem of death, psychoanalysts such as

Sanford (1957), Brodsky (1959), Norton (1963) and Roose (1969), all commented on the continued reluctance to deal with dying. All noted the ambiguity and ambivalence in human attitudes towards death. Usually people will readily admit that death is a necessary and inevitable outcome of life; we owe Nature a death and all are expected to repay the debt. In other words, death is always defined rationally as a natural and inescapable human fate. Unconsciously, however, this rational understanding of death is unacceptable, and—as Freud stated: "Im Unbewussten sei jeder von uns von seiner Unsterblichkeit uberzeugt." [In the unconscious, everyone of us is convinced of his own immortality.]

In the development of modern thanathology, special credit must also be given to Eissler, who in his classical study (1955), brought attention to the problem of the psychiatric treatment of patients approaching death. In this context Eissler also discussed the role of the psychiatrist himself. In addition to individual death, he also focused on reactions to the death of a loved one where ambivalence toward the dying person is a major issue. Moreover, Eissler discussed the problem of death of an enemy, where he saw a wish for destruction combined with the basic issue of hostility. Eissler also saw the ambivalent reaction to loss of human life as the first step toward the denial of reality, aspects of which he regarded as central to all death situations.

Weisman and Hackett (1961) have contributed to the clinical approach to understanding the dying process with a description of three aspects of the study of death: the impersonal death, the interpersonal death and the intrapersonal death. Impersonal death is devoid of any human element, as in the case of a pathologist or statistician for whom indifference or the irrelevance of the human factors allows or enhances a distance from the personal dimension of death.

The interpersonal aspect of death concerns three different levels: (1) observation of the death of others; (2) emotional participation in their dying process; and (3) emotional manifestations occurring with the actual arrival of death and cessation of life. Examinations of the interpersonal death situation reveal that ambivalent feelings may remain partly or totally latent on all three levels. This is related to the realization that the death of another reminds us that we are still alive. Thus, the death of another with whom we are in contact strongly influences the way one perceives one's self. The death of another warns us of our own mortality but at the same time brings home the powerful message that we have successfully avoided a basic threat to our own existence. Unconsciously, the primary narcissistic feeling of survival apparently plays a major role in the integrative and adaptive processes required to master the interpersonal death situation. Another's death is perceived as a personal challenge successfully met.

Intrapersonal death is the death of the individual himself. The narcissistic involvement in the death of another affirms that the intrapersonal or subjective aspects of death are the real core of the problem. This was the conclusion of Weisman and Hackett's (1961) study as well as those of Bromberg and Schilder (1936) and Eissler (1955).

Over many years as head of the psychiatric consultation service in a university teaching hospital, the author has had ample opportunity to become acquainted with problems of the dying patient, involving the patient himself and the reactions of his family and the professional staff to the dying person. Following acts of war and violence, it was possible to observe and study most situations which have been described by investigators in this field. The doctor-patient relationship with reference also to patients' families and physicians' attitude to fatal and malignant conditions was repeatedly examined and continuously emphasized to medical students and young resident physicians. In the course of this work, the need to extend our understanding of the processes revolving around the dying patient became imperative.

The Dying Process: Three Case Histories

Continued progress in this area depends on a better understanding of the process of denial as it develops in the dying patient, the family and in the physician himself. Proper evaluation of the process of denial enables a better therapeutic approach to the dying patient as well as to the family.

To illustrate, three cases involving malignant diseases and eventual death will be presented. Because the concept of ego-strength is a key aspect of the author's views, two of the descriptions will emphasize this aspect. The third case is entirely clinical and involves a patient who developed a malignant disease while undergoing psychoanalysis. Juxtaposition of material originating from two structurally different sources—conscious vs. unconscious—will be used to elucidate some theoretical issues involved in attitudes to death.

The first case is a father's story of his son's illness and untimely death. First published 30 years ago, John Gunther's *Death Be Not Proud* is a memoir of and tribute to his son Johnny, who died at 17, after a fifteen-month illness. The book contains excerpts from Johnny's own letters and diary during his illness and a short epilogue written by his mother.

The second case is that of the well-known American columnist, Stewart Alsop, who died of leukemia in 1974. In *Stay of Execution*, he describes the first 14 months of his illness and his reactions. It is a study of what it means to live with a terminal disease and to be confronted daily with the immediate prospect of one's own death.

Case History 1. Johnny Gunther died of a malignant brain tumor. The final diagnosis was multiple glioma. During the 15 months when he lived with the tumor, Johnny made excruciating efforts to pursue and attain goals he had set for himself before he was struck by the disease. These included completing high school and applying for acceptance to Harvard University. The prospect of a drastically shortened life apparently spurred him on to new and renewed involvement in his many fields of interest. Thus, during his illness, he completed 50 reports on chemical experiments he had performed, maintained correspondence with teachers and friends, and studied for (and passed) all his examinations—with an orange-sized tumor growing fatally in his brain. Reading the book, one receives the impression that Johnny refused to accept the fact that his world was vanishing. From the very beginning his parents were given detailed information about the nature of their son's illness. While they accepted the basic facts, they continued to deny the implications until the very moment of Johnny's death, which they reacted to with panic and a feeling "that his life departed covertly. Like a thief death took him."

A brave facade was kept up between Johnny and his parents. They never spoke about the shocking and frightening nature of Johnny's deteriorating condition. As his doctors were rather candid with him, Johnny was aware of his desperate condition. The non-communication between Johnny and his parents on this most central issue can be called an induction of denial, i.e., the development of a protective layer of denial through which the complicated emotional issues are treated. Gunther's book also reveals that Johnny became preoccupied with the relationship of his divorced parents as well as with trying to understand why their marriage had failed. As will be discussed later, this is of prime importance as it enabled him to strengthen old emotional attachments.

The parents' attitude toward the physicians reflected ambivalent feelings: on the one hand hope and appreciation, and on the other, hidden and even manifest anger. The positive feelings were maintained until the moment they realized that the physicians could not defeat the disease. This parental despair expressed itself at the final moment of death: "All the doctors—helpless flies now, climbing across the granite face of death."

Case History 2. Without the sentimentality of Gunther's book, Alsop's reflections are deeply moving. At the peak of his career, a 57-year-old, happily married man, the father of six children, suddenly realized that death is imminent. On the conscious level, this is the story of his uncertain medical diagnosis: Does he have acute myeloblastic leukemia or not? On the unconscious level, it is the story of flickering but persistent attempts to come to terms with the incredulous prospect of death. Alsop wrote: "I knew in my mind [on the day he learned the diagnosis] that I would almost certainly die quite soon, but in my heart I refused to believe it." His efforts at denial eventually resulted in "a kind of unhappy inner stolidity combined with a strong protective instinct that somebody else will die." Much of Alsop's book deals with incidents from his past, his formative years. It is clear that by dealing extensively with the past, Alsop sought to stabilize his perception of the present by tying the two as firmly together as possible. The future is touched upon only in terms of some indefinite period, the time he has left to life. In the context of his preoccupation with the past, Alsop's book describes a combination of partial regression coupled with a *counterphobic* mechanism which helped him to cope: the compulsive repetition of childhood prayers. Thus, fear and uncertainty about the future generated an unconscious preoccupation with the past.

To cope with the anxieties of the present, Alsop also developed a very strong attachment to his physician. It is as if he tried to push away his malignancy through the process of fighting it by knowing about it. Alsop learned the significance of his blood counts, cell types and marrow tests. Thus, he could in a sense, step away and impersonally observe the medical data as it oscillated between the extremes of life and death. Alsop and his physician communicated through this protective layer of medical terminology and blood count figures. This process of handling the complicated and frightening emotional issues through a common frame of reference, which decidedly did not include the implications of the facts discussed, represents the induction of denial.

With time, however, Alsop found it increasingly difficult to separate hard statistics from feelings and agreed with his physician that he would not be told the results of the crucial marrow test. When no promise was held in one quarter, he sought it in another. Eventually, however, promises became much less than believable and it appears that Alsop resolved to give up attempts at denial and instead try to make the best of life as long as possible. He wrote, "A dying man needs to die, as a sleepy man needs to sleep, and there comes a time when it is wrong, as well as useless, to resist."

Case History 3. While in analysis with the author, a patient developed an acute monocytic leukemia. After the onset of illness, analysis continued for one year until the time of death.

The patient, a 34-year-old highly intelligent woman, the mother of two sons, had been referred for therapy by a gynecologist, whom she had consulted about sexual difficulties with her husband. She presented with tension and mild depression.

Reluctant to undergo treatment, the patient was at first horrified at the idea of exposing herself in the analytic situation. In spite of these initial difficulties, however, she quickly developed an intense relationship with her analyst. At first, her psychological problems appeared to be of an hysterical nature. The oedipal conflict seemed to be of primary importance in her psychopathology. Her unconscious comparison of her husband with her father, whom she described as a strong, extroverted, lusty person, interfered with her sexual functioning.

Her therapy began in the accepted manner, with the evaluation of basic defense mechanisms such as regression. Initially the patient described her childhood as relatively unproblematic, but it was nonetheless clear that she had immigrated to Israel following marriage to break away from the family circle. Already the early phase of therapy revealed the obvious oedipal nature of her transference. The patient felt a very strong competition with her analyst's other patients and expressed her concern that she might be of less interest to him than others. Her needs to be cared for were examined and a fear of being rejected as well as a tendency to compete for love and attention were discussed.

At this stage in her therapy, very little mention had been made of her mother. Motherhood, however, was defined in positive terms, and she asserted that her children were her major satisfaction in life. The pregenital component of her difficulties nonetheless soon became clear. The preoedipal attachment to the mother, whom she described as overanxious, inhibited and unable to express emotions as well as the patient's father could, had brought her to a developmental fixation. The constellation of her difficulties, thus, was one in which the patient was unable to accept the mother role—as she had identified with the father in childhood. At the same time this left her with sexual inhibitions as she feared her mother's revenge. Presenting herself as a good mother manifested a tendency to overcompensation.

At this point it became clear that the main objective of therapy would be the solution of her conflicts with her mother. However, although the mother problem was central to her difficulties, the nature of transference still remained purely oedipal.

While claiming that she had made real efforts to succeed in therapy, the patient did not feel that the experience had fulfilled her expectations. She complained that the analyst's coldness toward her was the reason. She could only blame him for what she felt was lack of interest on his part. Despite her anger at the analyst, it was clear she hoped to influence him to change his attitude. In the following sessions she developed a different attitude in which the major issue was to display her ability to be a good mother. In this context, she expressed the hope of becoming pregnant and having more children. These developments assisted the patient in bringing up her sexual difficulties, and this quickly led her to deal with memory traces of her early relationship with her mother. For example, she related that she had always found it intolerable to be kissed. A kiss on the lips caused her anxiety and revulsion. She recalled that once as a teenager she had been kissed by a boyfriend, who had clumsily scratched her lips, causing her to bleed profusely. Her mother reproached her sternly for being kissed. It was around the seventh month of therapy that repressions about memories relating to her mother were partly lifted.

During the time that analysis focused more and more on her relationship with her mother, the patient became increasingly depressed. She came regularly to therapy, but complained of suffering from colds, fever and chilly sensations. Within a few weeks her weakness and pallor became prominent. She felt irritated with herself, blaming herself for being weak not only emotionally but also physically, and resolved to overcome her condition without the "idiotic pills" which had been prescribed by her family doctor.

About this time the patient reported a vivid dream wherein a preoccupation with death was present. In view of the developments which were to follow, it seems at least possible that this dream reflected a perception of those alarming body stimuli, the implications of which could be accepted neither by the unconscious nor the conscious. One could also claim that the analyst's concern for his patient's condition was reinforced by her unusual dream of death, thus causing him to perceive it as having special significance. Indeed, upon his urging, she agreed to consult an internist. A clinical examination and hospitalization eventually produced a diagnosis of monocytic leukemia.

This development raised questions about how to continue with therapy. At the patient's request—and in line with the analyst's considerations—it was decided that therapy would continue at least as many hours as before. Undoubtedly the process of induction of denial was present. Thus, when the patient asked her analyst if he knew of her diagnosis and he answered affirmatively, she indicated that she also knew it. Apart from that, they did not discuss the topic and its dire implications further. Because of the rapid approach of death, the analyst felt the patient would gain immensely if she could resolve her problems with her mother. The rationale was that a reinvestment into a good and long-desired emotional attachment with her mother would decrease the strain on her ego, thus strengthening it.

Therapy was apparently successful in accomplishing this. The patient's renunciation of her mother was first brought up to the conscious level in the context of how to care for her own children during her illness. She thought of inviting her mother to come and take care of them, and then realized that she herself did not want her mother's care, preferring that of her analyst instead. As painful as this insight was, it nonetheless showed that she was well on her way to accepting her own need for loving care from her mother. This final step was secured partly through interpretation of a dream which revealed that she did not want to show herself in her present deteriorated condition to her mother, and partly through working out the panic resulting from a severe hemmorrhage from the mucosa of the mouth, which brought back the memory of the teenage kiss. After this, the patient felt she had to see her mother. She died on the night of the day her mother arrived. The patient was calm and happy when she arrived and they spent her last few hours of life talking about her childhood.

The Problem of Denial

Drawing upon these three illustrations, a number of theoretical issues will be reviewed and discussed. It is clear that denial assumes a major role in the dying process and in confrontation with death. However, a reexamination of Anna Freud's definition of denial as by word, by act and by fantasy, makes it clear that the usual connotations of denial cannot be applied when dealing with the death situation. The problem with the previous definition of denial is that it pertains more to the ways and means by which an issue may be denied than to the issue which is denied itself. Thus, it may be said that the definition deals with the form in which contents are manipulated in the unconscious rather than with the contents which are manipulated.

The idea of death cannot be grasped by the unconscious, and thus the conflict does not even reach the unconscious level. Consequently the process of denial does not and cannot run its ordinary course. In the death situation, the unconscious simply does not provide material necessary for potential denial.

The process of denial can be explained on a level closer to the ego and can be better understood in terms of the interaction between the ego of the dying person and the social system reacting to the dying person. The social system may be a hospital where the person is hospitalized, it may be the family circle around the individual, or both. Before discussing these aspects, however, the missing link between Anna Freud's views of the mechanism of denial and those of the author must be filled in.

This link is the contribution of Weisman (1972) who has suggested a structural definition of denial including a progressive scale for its classification. Weisman proposed that the process of dying may be seen as a graduation of denial from a first order, through a second to a third order. The first order of denial relates to the mere facts of the illness only. The patient, in other words, denies the primary facts as well as symptoms of the illness, trying to believe that what he has is a much less severe disease with a favorable prognosis. There is little doubt that the analytic patient used this form of denial, even when experiencing severe physical symptoms. Alsop's preoccupation with the different diagnostic possibilities of his illness reflects the use of a similar mechanism.

The progress of the denial process is like falling back on second and third lines of defense. On the second order of denial, some basic facts about the illness are accepted, but their implications are denied. The patient does not reach any further conclusions about life and death in the context of the malignancy and its dictates. This kind of denial easily lends itself to description using the well-known entities of rationalization, avoidance and—at times—even displacement. Gunther's memoir relates many such instances. Thus, for example, even after a diagnosis has been made, Johnny's parents did not project its implications into the future. Rather, they believed that a diligent search would turn up a cure. Their last minute panic before Johnny died also attests to the presence of this type of denial.

The last line of defense is denial of the third order in which extinction itself is denied. This type of denial is in accordance with the earlier stated inability to relate to the idea of subjective death. As a characteristic and dominant form of denial, this type refers to the severely ill only. As a terminal disease advances, patients reach this stage generally after passing through the other two. Theoretically, however, all three levels of denial can be present at the same time. A discussion of the third form of denial will almost inevitably reveal considerable disagreement even among professionals, not to mention family members. This form of denial could be interpreted as a demonstration of ego strength but it may equally well be argued that what is revealed is religious faith or a combination of optimism and bravery. Surely other interpretations could be argued as well, all depending upon the particular metaphysical or spiritual outlook with which this form of denial is sought and integrated. John Gunther undoubtedly saw in his son an unusual measure of bravery and persistence in the pursuit of his goals.

Additional insight into the process of denial is gained by taking a somewhat more dynamic approach involving not only denial as a mechanism and its structured gradation as suggested by Weisman, but also the interaction between the patient and the surrounding social structure.

The dying person becomes increasingly desocialized. In this context, desocialized refers not to increasing personal disorganization, but to the fact that social interaction on the part of the dying person becomes increasingly limited, although it is conceivable that there will be cases in which the two occur together. How does this process start and from where does it derive its impetus? The healthy person who is active within his social system continuously multiplies his social roles. In contrast, the dying person is forced to limit his social roles and commitments. Moreover, either due to physical limitations imposed by the malignancy or because of its concomitant psychological manifestations, the patient gravitates towards somewhat more monolithic forms of behavior. This development, however, is matched by a reaction pattern in the surrounding social structure, and the interaction between them is one of mutual reinforcement.

The dying patient has an increased need to reinforce emotional relationships. Therefore, interpersonal factors involving the dying patient and his social environment intermingle with an unconscious current characterized by a both covert and overt search for emotional support. There is thus, in the dying patient, a susceptibility to grasp also unconscious messages emanating from his surrounding environment.

The "Induction of Denial": Discussion and Conclusion

This process may be viewed as the attempts of the dying person to hold on to reality in the face of growing desocialization imposed upon him by the progress of his disease. The susceptibility to grasp unconscious messages is reinforced by the environment and its members, who have their own unconscious attitudes to death. This results in a mutually beneficial unspoken agreement to deny the impending death. The unconscious denial by others in his environment precipitates and enhances the process of denial in the patient himself. This "induction of denial" is used by both the family of the dying person and his physicians as protection and defense on two levels: one corresponding to the satisfaction of their altruistic needs and the other one on which defenses are mobilized against the narcissistic injury emanating from the death situation.

The satisfaction of these needs goes hand in hand with the satisfaction of the needs of the dying person. Indeed, what does the dying person expect from his environment? Is he actually in quest of the truth about his illness? Does he really want to learn his final diagnosis or does he want to hear the opposite and a series of comforting lies? The case of the analytic patient indicates—as much as the other two histories—that these questions are of a secondary nature. The real issue behind them is the wish of the dying person to find or reinforce a basic trust in his vanishing world. This point is probably best illustrated in Alsop's work where he describes his struggle with the truth of his malignancy's progress. At one point he resolved with his physician that he would not be told the results of his vital blood counts, which until then had functioned as an erratic measuring rod of his doubtful prognosis. He would rather attempt to go on living and include his medical rigors in his daily routine. Clearly, Johnny's valiant struggle to fulfill school requirements and to proceed with his chemical experiments may be appreciated in this light, too.

It appears, therefore, that valuable support may be found for the dying if they can secure and rely upon a basic trust in the world. The question then becomes how to achieve this. An answer is suggested from a general structural psychoanalytic point of view and secondly from a dynamic therapeutic angle.

The process of dying undoubtedly includes the withdrawal of partial libidinal interest from other persons as well as from interests and activities. As previously mentioned, the progress of malignant disease is associated with decreased social interaction between the dying and his environment. The induction of denial engineered by the patient and the members of his environment is designed to counteract this process, but may well function as a protective layer with the overall result being an enhancement of the feeling of rejection. The dying patient most surely has to reinvest some of his freed libido in this process. In a sense, this is both made possible for him and demanded from him by those with whom he interacts.

However, as just seen, the induction of denial hardly functions to alleviate the underlying problem of establishing or preserving a basic trust in the world. If, on the other hand, fragments of the libidinal energy could be reinvested into old emotional attachments, one could expect a concurrent decrease of emotional threat caused by the growing loss of external reality. The reunion and "Liebstod" fantasies of the dying person therefore may be understood and interpreted as spontaneous attempts at redistribution of libidinal energy. Through the precipitation of regression along these lines to an earlier ego state, the need for cathexis should also be lessened. If this can be attained, the dying person may consequently be spared a painful psychological struggle, the overall result of the procedure being a relative strengthening of the ego.

Both the analytic patient and Stewart Alsop had recourse to this procedure. Alsop describes a combination of partial regression and counterphobic mechanisms, which he found helpful in coping with his anxieties. He also went back in his thoughts to draw out key aspects of the past, subsequently seeking to integrate them with the uncertain present. The analytic patient made a comparable regression through her relationship with her analyst and managed to rework her complicated relationship with her mother, undoubtedly much to her benefit despite the fact that she died very soon after accomplishing this.

The case of the analytic patient may be used to illustrate the problem of achieving basic trust in the world when viewed from the therapeutic angle. It has been suggested that the dying person may benefit from making a regression with reinvestment of libido into prior emotional attachments. If the dying person carries this out on his own, the process will often meet with severe obstacles because of unconscious emotional conflicts. If this happens, the patient may benefit from therapy. The question is then how should the therapist handle the situation. The central aspect in this context is the problem of transference and particularly countertransference. Physicians, as well as family members, are also prone to induce denial as part of their own unconscious reaction to death.

Even the very experienced and "forcedly impersonal, desensitized" physician is not unaffected when confronted with the impending death of another person. Norton (1963) defines this aspect of the doctor-patient relationship as "consciously accepted countertransference." The dying patient stimulates the doctor, therapist or psychoanalyst to encounter his own guilt feelings. A life that cannot be saved not only narcissistically wounds the physician's pride, but stirs up his own anxieties.

Forced to find their own ways to deal with this characteristic reaction, physicians often tend to withdraw, avoiding confrontation with the patient and escaping into a sometimes indiscriminate administration of sedatives and painkillers. It is a commonly observed phenomenon too that doctors on their rounds make only a perfunctory call on dying patients. This withdrawal from the dying patient is of course rationalized as consideration for family members, avoiding chances of infection or not disturbing the patient. But often this facade masks the physician's underlying feelings of guilt about his failure and his inability to tolerate a threat to his feelings of omnipotence. Such feelings are often responsible for the fact that dying patients are so frequently left to die alone. Doctors as well as families of dying patients defend themselves against these internal threats in ways varying from anxiety and guilt to anger or grief. Psychoanalysts claim that acceptance and awareness of those feelings may help one to avoid denial, repression and overprotection, or the unjustified optimism of the physician, which interferes with his ability to serve his patient's real needs. Apart from the workings of these complicated forces, there is little doubt that a physician's education has rather exclusively prepared him to try to save life, and not for the responsibility of dealing with dying and death.

In his paper on "Inhibition, Symptoms, and Anxiety" (1926), Freud wrote about the establishment of transference, meaning the mobilization of archaic trust in the world and the return to the experience of primordial feelings of being protected (by the mother). Eissler (1955) developed this idea further, claiming that by attaining such a feeling of archaic trust, the suffering of the dying person can be considerably reduced, even in the presence of extreme physical pain. Opinions vary as to how this trust is best established within the therapeutic situation. Eissler (1955) and Norton (1963) advocated the so-called "gift-situation," which is based on the theoretical concept that the therapist can and should offer himself as an available object for deep understanding and love. This attitude will be perceived by the patient as "an unusual favor of destiny," helping him to develop defenses against object loss. Others, like Roose (1969), justifiably refuse to accept this approach, as it implies that this type of love for the patient might take the form of pity and sorrow.

This writer objects to Eissler's and Norton's formulation on the grounds that this approach leaves much room for poorly-handled transference and largely unresolved countertransference problems. It also implies distorted reality perception on the part of the physician. When this is perceived by the dying person, it will most likely only undermine his will to trust in the world, which is increasingly represented only by his closest environment. As already noted, a different approach is suggested, based on Freud's notion that as libidinal interest and investment is withdrawn from a love object into the ego, it is followed by a damming up of libido. The therapist's task, therefore, is to assist the dying patient to redistribute this excess libido and to remove those emotional obstacles which prevent the dying person from making a meaningful reinvestment in old emotional attachments. The problem of countertransference should be dealt with, in this context, as an integral part of the treatment situation. The better this aspect is handled, the better is the treatment for the dying patient. The induction of denial, in both the patient and the therapist, must be faced and dealt with in the clinical situation.

Summary

Psychological data originating from conscious and unconscious sources in terminal patients were discussed. Interaction between the dying patient and members of his environment was examined. The paper emphasized that the central process of denial cannot be adequately accounted for by focusing exclusively upon the psychodynamics of the dying person. The concept of "induction of denial" was presented, and causes and consequences of it were critically examined.

"Induction of denial" seems to be an integral part of the therapeutic situation with terminal patients. It is argued that redistribution of libidinal energy including reinvestment into old emotional attachments might be considered of therapeutic value. Relative strengthening of the ego may ease the dying person's confrontation with death.

References

Alsop, S. *Stay of execution.* Philadelphia: Lippincott, 1973.
Brodsky, B. Liebestod fantasies in a patient faced with a fatal illness. *International Journal of Psychoanalysis,* 1959, *40,* 13.
Bromberg, W., & Schilder, P. The attitude of psychoneurotics towards death. *Psychoanalytic Review,* 1936, *23,* 1.

Eissler, K. R. *The psychiatrist and the dying patient.* New York: International University Press, 1955.

Freud, S. (Ed.). *The theme of the three caskets.* London: Hogarth Press, 1913, *12*, 289.

Freud, S. (Ed.). *Thought for the times on war and death.* London: Hogarth Press, 1915, *14*, 273.

Freud, S. (Ed.). *Inhibitions, symptoms and anxiety.* London: Hogarth Press, 1926, *20*, 87.

Gunther, J. *Death be not proud.* New York: The Modern Library, 1953.

Norton, J. Treatment of a dying patient. *Psychoanalytic Study of the Child,* 1963, *18*, 541.

Roose, L. J. The dying patient. *International Journal of Psychoanalysis,* 1969, *50*, 385.

Sanford, B. Some notes on a dying patient. *International Journal of Psychoanalysis,* 1957, *38*, 158.

Schur, M. *Freud: living and dying.* New York: International University Press, 1972.

Troup, S. P., & Greene, W. A. *The patient, the death and the family.* New York: Charles Scribner's Sons, 1974.

Weisman, A. D. *On dying and denying.* New York: Behavior Books, 1972.

Weisman, A. D., & Hackett, T. P. Predilection to death: Death and dying as a psychiatric problem. *Psychosomatic Medicine,* 1961, *23*, 231.

Section III
❖
Mind-Body Interactions and Their Impact on Life-Threatening Illness

11

Grief, Immunity and Morbidity: Psychophysiological Interactions

Roger Bartrop, Ronald Penny, Michael Jones, Lina Forcier

Introduction

The past decade has witnessed intensified scientific interest in the hypothesized links between potentially stressful life events and health within the now commonly accepted multicausal theories of disease. A large number of current research initiatives are directed towards measuring changes in an individual's environment, especially those demanding changes having personal significance, with a view to examining whether such events are linked to disease.

Bereavement is generally accepted to be one of the most stressful life events (Tennant & Andrews, 1976), and as such is a good model for assessing the possible physiological and psychological impacts of a stress event. It can be readily identified objectively (Weiner, Note 1; Bartrop & Porritt, 1988). It can easily be dated and it has substantial effects on mood and behavior. It is distinct from other adverse life events in that it is not an effect of any pre-existing disturbance in the bereaved and it is unlikely to be confounded with physical or psychiatric illness. Moreover, almost all individuals encounter the experience and some do so more than once. There are, however, several problems such as the impracticality of obtaining baseline data and the difficulty of dating precisely the onset of the stress when there is prior warning of bereavement.

It has been hypothesised that perturbations of the immune system could be the intermediate link in the pathogenesis between stressor(s) and particular diseases. Bahnson (1981) has postulated that amplification and sustained production of the heterogeneous neuropeptide hormones could be important hormonal bridges between emotional states and the complex lymphocyte activity in many neoplastic diseases. The author's project (described below) represented one of the early attempts to use bereavement stress to provide some of the answers to the questions raised by such postulates of a biopsychosocial model of disease.

Stress and immune dysfunction

There is already evidence that various chronic stressors can result in dysfunction of the immune system. Kiecolt-Glaser and Glaser (1986) have reported results from a cross-sectional study of marital dysharmony which showed that women who had separated from their husbands within the previous year had significantly poorer immune function and higher antibody titres to the Epstein Barr virus (EBV) than demographically matched married women. The significance of short-lasting life events implicating chronic difficulties was exemplified by studies showing a decline (compared to baseline) in natural killer (NK) cell activity in final year medical students one month prior to and during the stressful final examinations (Kiecolt-Glaser et al, 1984). The more lonely students had significantly lower NK levels. These data were reproduced in two other samples (Kiecolt-Glaser et al, 1986, Glaser et al, 1986).

Stress, immune dysfunction and cancer

The psychosomatic literature over the past half century has highlighted the anecdotal and empirical evidence purporting to document the centuries-old truism that the inability to express emotion may be involved in cancer onset and progression. In recent years, seemingly paradoxical findings have begun to accrue about coping styles and breast cancer progression, a better prognosis being associated with women expressing hostile, anxious and assertive affect (previously often labelled 'negative affects').

Landmark research by British workers (Greer and Morris, 1975; Pettingale et al., 1977) with non-structured interviews and, more recently, the development of the Cortauld Emotional Control Scale by Greer's group (Watson and Greer, 1983), as well as data coming from replication studies by Scherg, Cramer and Blohmke (1981) and Wirsching et al. (1982), have enabled such an accrual of convergent findings that the notion of a type 'C' cancer-prone individual has been developed (characterized by suppressed anger, unassertiveness and the exhibition of conformity and compliance).

Extensions of the above work have been reported by Levy et al. (1985) and Dean and Surtees (1989) where distress and maladjustment prior to or at the time of breast cancer surgery was correlated with less frequent nodal involement and higher NK cell activity levels at follow-up.

Preliminary results from an Australian study (O'Donnell, 1992) support Levy et al.'s findings. Early breast cancer patients rated as poorly adjusted had significantly higher levels of NK cell activity. Although there was no replication of Levy et al.'s finding of higher NK cell activity in patients with no nodal involvement, the Australian group did demonstrate significantly higher scores on the Cortauld Emotional Control Suppression of Anger sub-scale in patients with nodal involvement compared with those with no nodal involvement. A significant inverse correlation between beta endorphin and NK cell activity in mastectomy but not lumpectomy patients indicated some of the neuro-regulatory pathways that may be involved in the mediation of psychosocial effects.

Pettingale (1985) has cautioned that any attempt to prove the importance of psychological factors in the development of human tumors may be unsuccessful owing to the considerable biological heterogeneity of such pathology. However, once such tumors are diagnosed, it may be possible at least to discover whether patients with suppression of anger exhibit a (postulated) augmented or prolonged hormonal response, and further to examine whether these patients are more vulnerable in terms of diminished survival time.

Stress, immune dysfunction, and mortality

The possible relationship between stress, the immune system and subsequent mortality also needs examination. There are examples where a stressor, such as bereavement, is associated with a higher mortality rate among spouse bereaved. Schleifer et al. (1983) and Lynch (1979) appear to attribute a significant proportion of spouse bereaved mortality to desolation and loneliness, but it is not clear, in the current state of our knowledge, that desolation or loneliness contributes alone, or even in large part, to the increased mortality rate in the newly widowed spouses (Young, Benjamin & Wallis, 1963; Cox & Ford, 1964; Helsing, Szklo & Comstock, 1981). Assortative mating in couples who both die early, a disadvantageous shared environment (in terms of living conditions), shared habits such as poor nutrition, poor exercise pattern, deleterious cigarette and alcohol consumption, and poor compliance with prescribed medication could all contribute to increased mortality rates in the first year of bereavement (Bartrop & Porritt, 1988). Further, a high incidence of death due to cardiovascular and cerebrovascular disease, and suicide are found in bereaved spouses. Some authors (for example, Maddox, 1984) query the relevance of such causes of death to a postulated immune system dysfunction in bereaved spouses.

In summary, studies over the last 15 years have given support to the theory that stressful life events can lead to increased morbidity and mortality. More research is required to gain a detailed understanding of the mechanisms involved. This chapter presents one project conducted in this area of research.

The Sydney, Australia, Bereavement Project (1975-1991)

Background

In 1975, a research team was formed from the staff of three Sydney, Australia, teaching hospitals to investigate putative associations between bereavement and physiological and psychological responses. The research project comprised three interrelated studies conducted between 1975-1991 with bereaved individuals and matched controls. Using bereavement as a model life event, the project was undertaken:

1) to clarify underlying factors involved in the aetiology of disease,

2) to gain a better understanding of the pathogenesis of various major causes of morbidity and mortality, and,

3) ultimately, to be able to use this information in the practice of preventive medicine (and, as a corollary, decrease long term health costs).

Study 1 (1975) examined immediate and intermediate immunological and endocrinological responses to the stressor. The aim was to test whether bereavement was associated with immunosuppression as measured by cellular (T cell function) and humoral (B cell function) immunity, and whether such immunosuppression was mediated by hypersecretion of hormonal factors such as thyroid hormones, cortisol, dopamine and serotonin.

Study 2 (1976-1977) was designed to explore further those tests of immunological and endocrinological function that had proven to be sensitive laboratory correlates of bereavement in Study 1. In addition, the second study incorporated psychosocial measures both at two weeks and six months following bereavement, so that interactions between these and the immunological and endocrinological functions could be examined.

Study 3 (1985-1991) re-enrolled the 1975 to 1977 subjects of both Studies 1 and 2 and examined their physical and psychiatric morbidity and mortality until December, 1985. It aimed to examine long-term effects (8-11 years) after bereavement on physical and psychological morbidity and mortality.

Only salient points of the methodology and results of Study 1 and Study 2 will be listed here, since most of that work has been described elsewhere (Bartrop et al., 1977; Bartrop & Porritt, 1988; Bartrop et al., 1992). Methodology and some results for Study 3 are also given here.

Study 1 (1975)

This study examined possible immunological disturbances following bereavement, and investigated the possibility of these disturbances being mediated by hormonal changes.

Methods

Bereaved subject group. Thirty-four individuals in good health whose spouse or close relative had died as a result of injury or illness in one of the three participating hospitals, agreed to be enrolled in the study within one week of their bereavement. Twenty-six of the bereaved subjects between the ages of 20 and 65 years gave blood for the detailed laboratory analyses. The upper age limit was imposed because of the T cell function changes with age (Foad et al., 1974). Counseling was offered to those individuals who needed it.

Control subject group. One community volunteer or hospital staff control, matched for sex and age and who had not been bereaved in the previous two years, was selected for each bereaved subject. The 26 controls, whose matched bereaved cases had venepuncture, also gave blood for laboratory measurements.

Laboratory tests and other data collected. Table 1 summarizes the procedures involved in Study 1. The study was explained to the subject at the first meeting. Further contact was maintained with all families either directly or through ministers of religion or social workers.

Each of the 34 bereaved subjects and their controls were interviewed. The questionnaire included *socio-demographic*

Table 1
Summary of Procedures
Study 1 (a "+" denotes time at which data collection occurred)

VISIT NUMBER	1	2	3	4	5	6	7
PERIOD SINCE BEREAVEMENT	—	14 days	16 days	4 weeks	8 weeks	average 5 months	6 months
DATA OBTAINED							
Sociodemographic	+						
Life events and personality scales						+	
Medical history	+						
Blood collected and laboratory tests conducted							
• T cell function	+				+		+
• delayed hypersensitivity	+	+					
• B cell function	+			+			
• T cell numbers	+				+		
• B cell numbers	+				+		
• Hormonal assays	+				+		
• Autoantibodies	+						
• Serum proteins	+				+		
• Alpha 2-macroglobulins	+				+		

variables such as: the matching variables (age, and sex); quality and length of marriage; occupational status of the subject and the deceased was coded using Congalton's (1969) four-point scale for occupational prestige; religion; the number of first degree relatives and the quality of their help; the number of close friends and their perceived helpfulness. Because these variables could have been associated with blood biochemistry changes, and may have been differentially distributed in the bereaved and the controls, they were potential confounders and so needed to be controlled for in the analysis of the data.

Data concerning other potential confounders were also collected. Several measures of personality function were used: The State Trait Anxiety Scale (STAI) (Spielberger, Gorsuch & Lushene, 1970) and the Affiliation, Autonomy, and Social

Desirability Scales from the Jackson Research Form (Jackson, 1967). The Tennant and Andrews Life Event Inventory was also employed (1976). Further, for the bereaved, the period between expectancy of death and its occurrence was recorded and classified on a five point scale from less than 24 hours to over three months warning.

Subjects with haematological, immunological, or allergic disorders in the preceeding two years were excluded after examination of their medical history. Exclusion criteria were: blood dyscrasias, autoimmune disease, immune deficiency states and allergies; subjects who had received a booster tetanus injection or a full course of tetanus toxoid within the previous five years; subjects with recent or current drug regimens including known or presumed immunosuppressants. Other information was also obtained: a history of specific drug treatment for depression during the six months of the study and a history of prior treatment for psychiatric disorder and its management (whether inpatient, outpatient or non-specialist).

For logistical reasons, the endocrinological and immunological variables could be collected in only a sample of the study subjects. Of the 34 controls and 34 bereaved cases, 26 controls and 26 matched bereaved cases had blood samples taken at the same time for identical laboratory testing. The laboratory tests performed included:

1) a lymphocyte transformation test using the mitogens phytohaemagglutinin (PHA) and concanavalin (Con A), and a test of delayed hypersensitivity as measures of T cell function (Bartrop et al., 1977);

2) an assessment of tetanus toxoid antibody levels following a tetanus toxoid challenge, and an assessment of serum immunoglobin levels (A, G and M), as measures of B cell function (Nelson, 1973; Bartrop et al., 1977);

3) the production of E and EAC rosette-forming lymphocytes as measures of T and B cell numbers, respectively, as well as a total lymphocyte count as a measure for the T cell numbers, and surface membrane immunoglobulin as a further measure of B cell numbers (Cooper et al., 1975);

4) estimation of alpha 2-macroglobulin as a possible immunosuppressive effect on blastogenesis (Cooperband, 1974);

5) serum hormone assays: cortisol, triiodothyronine (T3), thyroxine (T4), dopamine and serotonin as possible intermediate links to explain any demonstrable disturbance of the immune system (Mason, 1972; Bartrop et al., 1977).

In addition, to ensure the exclusion or adjustment in the analysis of subjects entering the study suffering from immunological problems, investigations for autoantibodies were carried out. Nutrition as a possible confounder for immunological disturbances was measured using serum protein estimations.

Statistical analysis. Some data attrition occurred, and to retain as many data as possible in the analysis, unpaired analyses were performed instead of paired analyses. Unpaired t-tests were used except for the analysis of the categorical data of the delayed-type hypersensitivity test which was analyzed using the Fisher exact test (Siegal, 1956).

The initial analysis (Bartrop et al., 1977) of the T cell function data used the non-parametric Wilcoxon Sum Rank Test (WSRT) or the Mann-Whitney Test for non-paired data. The non-parametric analysis was similar to that used for other data in our laboratory at St. Vincent's Hospital and reflected that these measurements were not normally distributed. Ziegler, Hansen, and Penny (1975) developed a suitable transformation to normality allowing the more powerful t-test to be used. The results obtained for these data were similar regardless of which statistical analysis method was used.

Results

Interview data for the subjects of Study 1 combined with those of Study 2 are summarized in Table 3. The results of the laboratory tests are presented here.

Of the 52 subjects (26 bereaved and 26 controls) who gave blood, all autoantibody investigations were normal on entry into the study, so that no study subject had to be excluded because of pre-existing immunological disturbances. Further, the bereaved and non-bereaved subjects did not differ significantly on nutrition as measured by the serum protein investigations. Nutrition has been claimed to be a possible confounder for immunological dysfunction, and so could have hidden any effect of bereavement.

Bartrop et al. (1977) found that the only immunological test which differentiated between the bereaved and control groups was the T cell function test, i.e., the lymphocyte transformation test using the mitogens PHA and Con A. The bereaved showed a statistically significantly depressed immunological response overall at two weeks, eight weeks, and at six months. This depression was not always observed for the same mitogen stimulation at the same dose. By six months, the difference was statistically significant only with one dose of Con A mitogen.

There were no statistically significant differences between the bereaved and control groups for:

1) T cell function as measured by delayed-type hypersensitivity
2) B cell function
3) T and B cell numbers
4) Alpha 2-macroglobulin levels
5) Hormonal assays. Serum cortisol levels of the bereaved were higher than those of the controls, but not statistically significantly so.

Study 2 (1976-1977)

This study focused on the psychosocial outcome of bereavement by exploring the relationships between affective states and bereavement at both two weeks and six months after bereavement. It was postulated that the effects of bereavement on such outcome measures decline with time to a greater extent for some individuals than for others. Further, it was hypothesized that certain covariates would determine the six months outcome. This study also attempted another investigation of the endocrinological and immunological outcomes of bereavement.

Methods

Bereaved subject group. Sixty-eight bereaved subjects were enrolled within one week of bereavement. In Study 2, 60 study subjects were spouse bereaved and eight were bereaved of other immediate family members. Thirty-six bereaved subjects between the ages of 20 and 65 years gave blood for the laboratory tests.

Table 2
Summary of Procedures
Study 2 (a "+" denotes time at which data collection occurred)

VISIT NUMBER	1	2	3	4	5	6
PERIOD SINCE BEREAVEMENT	—	14 days	4 weeks	8 weeks	average 5 months	6 months
DATA OBTAINED						
Sociodemographic		+				
Life events and personality scales					+	
Medical history		+				
Affective response scales		+				+
Blood collected for various immunological and hormonal tests		+	+	+		

Control subject group. Sixty-eight control subjects from hospital staff and members of community service clubs were selected and matched to the bereaved subjects as in Study 1. Of these, the 36 controls whose matched bereaved subjects had a venepuncture, also gave blood for laboratory measurements.

Laboratory tests and other data collected. Table 2 presents the procedures used in Study 2. For all subjects (68 bereaved cases and 68 non-bereaved controls) all potential confounders investigated in Study 1 were examined. These were sociodemographic data, measurements of personality function and life event details over the two year period preceding bereavement. Subjects were screened again by means of a medical history to ensure the exclusion of those subjects with haematological, immunological and allergic disorders. The method of data collection was identical in both studies.

Psychosocial responses (affective responses) to bereavement were examined as outcome variables. Response was measured with four affect scales: Spielberger's STAI (State Trait Anxiety Inventory) (Spielberger Gorsuch & Lushene, 1970; Porritt & Bartrop, 1985), Hamilton depression scale (Hamilton, 1960), a list of grief-related symptoms (Bartrop et al., in press) and the Templer Death Anxiety Scale (Templer, 1970).

New methodology for the endocrinological and immunological tests was chosen in this study. The start of Study 2 in 1976 coincided with the planned start of a National Collaborative Leukemia Study, and the same laboratory personnel in the immunology laboratory were to perform tests in both this bereavement study and the Leukemia Study. For logistic reasons, only the T cell function and B function tests were conducted. Testing for T cell function was modified from that used in Study 1 although the B cell test was identical. Only serum cortisol tests were repeated in Study 2, using the same assay as in Study 1.

Statistical analysis. Differences in affective responses between bereaved and non-bereaved at two weeks and six months were analyzed using a two-way Multivariate Analysis of Variance (MANOVA). Only 55 spouse bereaved and their 55 controls were analyzed for affective response, as some data attrition occurred. Adjustment for co-variates, which could be potential confounders, was done using the same statistical technique.

Results

Table 3 summarizes the potential confounders for the outcome measures in Studies 1 and 2. Data for all 204 subjects in both studies are shown classified by bereavement status

Table 3
List of Potential Confounders
From Studies 1 and 2, by Sex and Bereavement Status

		MALE		FEMALE	
POTENTIAL CONFOUNDER	MEASURE	Bereaved (N=36)	Control (N=36)	Bereaved (N=66)	Control (N=66)
SOCIO-DEMOGRAPHIC					
Age	Mean	49.1	47.1	48.4	46.5
	S.D.	13.8	11.9	11.9	12.3
Relationship adjustment	Mean	0.4	0.1	0.8	0.5
	S.D.	0.9	0.5	1.0	1.0
Length of relationship	Mean	22.1	19.3	22.0	17.6
	S.D.	12.5	10.9	11.6	11.2
Finances	Mean	3.4	4.4	2.6	3.8
	S.D.	1.6	0.9	1.5	1.2
Occupation	Mean	2.9	2.2	3.0	2.6
	S.D.	0.8	0.9	0.9	0.8
Religion	Mean	0.6	0.6	0.4	0.5
	S.D.	0.9	0.9	0.8	0.8
Number of relatives	Mean	4.8	4.9	4.8	4.9
	S.D.	2.5	2.6	2.4	2.7
Relatives' help	Mean	3.8	4.0	3.2	3.9
	S.D.	2.6	2.3	2.2	2.5
Number of friends	Mean	5.4	7.1	6.5	4.9
	S.D.	4.0	4.5	5.5	3.9
Friends' help	Mean	4.1	5.0	4.3	3.4
	S.D.	2.6	3.2	3.9	2.7
PERSONALITY MEASURES					
Spielberger trait	Mean	36.7	33.3	39.1	34.8
	S.D.	12.1	7.1	10.5	9.3
Affiliation	Mean	14.4	15.2	14.2	15.7
	S.D.	4.1	2.8	3.5	2.8
Autonomy	Mean	7.7	7.6	5.9	6.7
	S.D.	3.4	3.1	2.6	3.3
Social desirability	Mean	16.3	17.0	15.4	16.9
	S.D.	2.9	1.6	3.1	2.0

and sex. Finances and occupation were found to be highly significantly different between bereaved and non-bereaved. Some other variables were also found to be differentially distributed between groups: relationship adjustment, length of relationship, and some of the personality measures. The differences found in these latter variables could be related to socioeconomic status or could be due to the effects of bereavement.

Affective responses to bereavement were examined among Study 2 subjects. The Hamilton scale did show statistically significant differences between bereaved and non-bereaved two weeks after bereavement (i.e., the bereaved were a depressed population), but not on the repeat measure at six months. The Spielberger STAI state measure showed that, at both two weeks and six months, distress scores were significantly higher for the bereaved when compared with the non-bereaved. The levels of distress observed in the bereaved were similar to those reported in psychiatric patients (Spielberger, Gorsuch & Lushene, 1970). Distress as measured with the grief-related symptoms check list also showed a similar pattern to the results obtained with the Spielberger STAI. There was no statistically significant difference in the scores on the Templer Death Anxiety scale between the bereaved and control groups on either occasion of testing. This scale therefore appeared to measure a stable dimension about death anxiety, independent of bereavement.

The analyses of the 55 bereaved and their matched controls revealed that financial status was related to the four mood measures used. However, when the analysis of outcome at six months was controlled for financial status as a covariate, the differences in mood scores were still statistically significant.

Study 2 used some laboratory techniques to measure immunological outcomes which were variations on those of Study 1. Unfortunately, changes in technique resulted in an absence of interpretable T cell data. The B cell function test did not show any statistically significant differences between bereaved and controls. The serum cortisol assays did show higher levels in the bereaved but these were not statistically significant.

Study 3 (1985-1987)

The aim of Study 3 was to study the potential long-term effects of bereavement on morbidity and mortality of the bereaved population, with a view to suggesting appropriate management at the onset of bereavement in the wider community if long-term problems were found in this study.

Methods

Follow-up. All subjects from both Study 1 and Study 2 were considered for re-enrolment, i.e., 102 bereaved (34 from Study 1 and 68 from Study 2) and 102 controls (34 from Study 1 and 68 from Study 2). Extensive tracking facilities were available via diaries of the 1975-77 periods, as well as assistance from other sources such as the Commonwealth Electoral Commission and the Deaths Section of the Registry of Births, Deaths and Marriages. Ultimately, a record was obtained of 199 of the original subjects living in Australia. Further, Australian sources also provided details about subjects in Britain, Germany and the USA. Only two subjects were not located—one woman living in Britain and another woman known to be living in Sydney. Thus 202 out of the original sample of 204 subjects were located. Results of the follow-up work are shown in Table 4, which also presents numbers of re-enrolled subjects in Study 3.

In the last 15 years, with advances in epidemiological study designs and improved understanding of bereavement, it has become increasingly evident that it is preferable to study well defined study factors and that spouse bereavement may differ from other types of bereavement. Consequently, although Study 3 data were collected on all re-enrolled study subjects, only those relating to spouse bereavement were analyzed and are presented here.

Study subject population. From Studies 1 and 2, there were 77 spouse bereaved and 86 control subjects re-enrolled in the study. Of these, five spouse bereaved and six controls had died.

Table 4
Studies 1 and 2 Subjects Follow-up and Re-enrollment of Study Subjects for Study 3

	Numbers of						
	Bereaved of			Controls matched to bereaved of			
	Spouse	Other	Total	Spouse	Other	Total	Matched pairs of subjects
ORIGINAL NUMBERS (paired)							
Study 1	30	4	34	30	4	34	
Study 2	59	9	68	59	9	68	
Total	89	13	102	89	13	102	102
FOLLOW-UP							
Lost	1	1*	2	1	1*	2	
Contacted	88	12	100	88	12	100	
STUDY 3 RE-ENROLLMENT							
Refused	9	2	11	1	—	1	
Total agreed	77	11	88	86	12	98	86
Alive	72	11	83	80	11	91	
Dead	5	—	5	6	1	7	

* 1 bereaved subject had feigned bereavement. Although this subject was traced, for the purpose of this work, the subject and his control are lost to follow-up.

Data Collected and Laboratory Tests Conducted.

Dead subjects. Details of deceased subjects were verified from the death certificates provided by the Deaths Section of the Registry of Births, Deaths, and Marriages, Sydney. ICD-9 codes were used to classify the cause of death.

Living subjects. A general questionnaire was administered by interviewers to each of the 163 re-enrolled study subjects. This questionnaire measured socio-economic status, health variables such as weight, smoking and drinking, details about other bereavements over the period of follow-up, financial status and details of long-term medication. For the bereaved only, the questionnaire asked about recurring unpleasant thoughts related to the original bereavement.

In the interview with both bereaved and non-bereaved, mood scales were administered. These included the Spielberger STAI anxiety state and trait scales, and the Hamilton Depression scale, as well as a self-report depression symptom scale from the Center for Epidemiologic Studies, Yale University, known as the CES-D (Radloff, 1977).

Morbidity outcome to December, 1985, as recalled by the subjects, was collected with the aid of a modified version of the health questionnaire used by the Australian Veterans' Health Studies (1984). Self-reported morbidity data were collected according to the year of occurrence, specific note being taken of disease states occurring on more than one occasion in the same year, and over several time periods. Disease descriptions were coded using ICD-9 (World Health Organization, 1977).

Morbidity data were also collected from medical records from various sources. This has been termed "record" morbidity for the purpose of discrimination from the "self-report" morbidity data collected from the subject. Morbidity data which matched in both the "self-report" source and the "record" source have been termed "confirmed." To ensure consistent data collection, the same questionnaire was completed as that used with the study subjects. Of the 163 surviving subjects consenting to be re-enrolled, only one subject refused to allow the principal investigator access to her medical records. All other subjects signed a consent form for permission to access medical information from records of their general practitioner(s) (GP), specialist(s) (SP) and hospital records (HR). After completion of this form, the GPs and, when possible, the consultants involved, were contacted. Hospital records were also sought. Collection of morbidity data involved examination of records from over 500 doctors.

Among control subjects three were reported as having no illness by any of the sources while all bereaved subjects had at least one illness episode. The maximum number of illnesses recorded per subject was 20 for one bereaved subject, and 23 for one non-bereaved subject.

The method of interview (for both subject and the doctors) was recorded either as a clinical meeting, a telephone call, correspondence, or a combination of these methods. The number of doctors seen by the subject and the number of visits to general practitioners over the follow-up period were also recorded.

In addition, subjects were tested for T cell subsets and function (blastogenesis). Further details about these methodologies and results of data analyses will be included in a later report.

Statistical analysis. The data were entered into computer files and analyzed using BMDP (Dixon et al., 1990) and SPIDA (McNeil & Lunn, 1988). Frequency cross-tabulation and other descriptive measures were generated using BMDP.

Log-linear regression was used to analyze mortality and morbidity rates (Breslow et al., 1983). This form of analysis examines the association between bereavement and mortality/morbidity but takes into account the period for which subjects were at risk in the study. Relative risk estimates, obtained from the log-linear regression models provide a quantitative measure of the mortality and morbidity rates of bereaved subjects compared with controls.

Results

Over the eleven-year period, the spouse-bereaved subjects experienced a higher rate of morbidity compared to the non-bereaved control group (Table 5). This elevation is greater than can be attributed to chance according to any of the three sources reported.

Differences were found between bereaved and non-bereaved subjects for their distribution of occupational, financial and medication-related variables. Analyses which adjusted for these variables as well as a number of other variables were performed.

With the morbidity data obtained from the self and record reports, none of the potentially confounding factors explained the effect of bereavement. That is, after controlling for these factors individually, the difference between bereaved and controls was still statistically significant for both sources. In

Table 5
Summary of Relative Morbidity Rates for Bereaved Compared with Non-Bereaved at Full Follow-Up Time
(unadjusted data)

Morbidity Data Source	Illness-Score[4]		Relative Morbidity Rate	95% Conf. Interval	p-value
	Bereaved	Non-Bereaved			
Self-Report[1]	1439	1133	1.4	1.3, 1.5	<0.0001
Record[2]	1359	1181	1.3	1.2, 1.4	<0.0001
Confirmed[3]	620	542	1.3	1.1, 1.4	<0.0001

1 – as obtained from study subject
2 – as obtained from general practitioner(s), specialist(s) or hospital records
3 – as found in both the self-report and record sources
4 – results are based on illness-score, not only the number of illnesses. A subject's illness score was defined as the number of years for which their medical history was available, for a given source, during the time frame of the study.

the case of confirmed reports, several factors appear to confound the difference between bereaved and controls although most of these factors (such as medication use and marital status) are arguably outcomes rather than true confounding factors.

An analysis was made of the ICD-9 categories contributing to the elevation of the bereaved subjects' illness scores. At twelve months, two years and full follow-up time, several diseases in the circulatory and mental categories were more common among the bereaved. At full follow-up time, other ICD-9 categories (such as endocrine, nutritional and metabolic, injury, digestive, respiratory, and musculoskeletal) showed a significant increase in the bereaved in one or more data sources. The cancer rate, apart from some mis-classified solar keratoses in the self-report data source, showed no real increase when doctors' data cards were examined.

Mortality

The number of deaths in each study group was small, too small in fact for a meaningful conclusion to be drawn.

Discussion and Future Tasks

Since the work conducted in Study 1, another research group has confirmed depression of mitogen-stimulated T cell responsiveness in bereaved subjects (Schleifer et al., 1983). It, therefore, seems that a potential stressor such as bereavement can lead to perturbation of the immune system. Study 2 data showed that spouse bereaved individuals were more distressed when compared with non-bereaved, and many of the former suffered depression to a clinical degree. A population of bereaved could, therefore, concurrently exhibit psychological as well as immunological disturbances. Unfortunately, the change in blastogenesis technique (T cell function) in Study 2 invalidated any attempt to correlate disturbances in emotional state and in T cell function as outcome measures in the same individuals. There is research which can substantiate a potential association, for example, disturbances in T cell function in anxiety states (Linn, Linn & Jenson, 1981) and during episodes of endogenous depression (Schleifer et al., 1984; Schleifer et al., 1985; Kronfol et al., 1986; Irwin et al., 1990). Schleifer and co-workers (1984, 1985) concluded that altered lymphocyte function was more specific to the severe depressive symptoms expected in inpatient populations than in outpatients, other psychiatric populations or in groups hospitalized for the treatment of other pathology.

The link between endocrine and immune system changes was not established in Study 1 which tested for this potential connection. The Australian group as well as North-American and European research teams are examining the possible immunosuppresive role of the heterogeneous family of neuropeptides produced by the hypothalamo-pituitary axis as well as other neuro-regulatory pathways.

It is prudent to remember that when one deals with measurements from several frames of reference such as at the emotional, neuroendocrinological and immunological levels, it may be inappropriate to imply that one variable influences the other in a linear fashion, for all may reflect different aspects of the same basic process. The question of inherited predisposition also needs addressing. For example, in studies in which an association between anger suppression and development of breast cancer was found (Greer & Watson, 1985), it is possible that predisposition to both emotional inhibition and susceptibility to the development of cancer result from the individual's genetic constitution.

More prospective studies are needed to examine all aspects of individuals at high risk of morbidity and mortality following stressful circumstances. Study 3 is one such study. It followed up the health experiences over eight to eleven years of bereaved subjects who, in earlier psychoimmunological research, had exhibited transient immunosuppression extending over several months following their bereavement. Other research is also supportive of associations between changes to the immune system and long-term morbidity. There is evidence for a relationship between immunosuppression following transplant surgery and the development of a variety of common cancers in the recipients, often many years after transplantation (Sheil, 1987).

From our preliminary data it would appear that life crises such as bereavement increases physical and psychiatric morbidity rates, and may lead to increases in the use of medical services (Mechanic, 1980). Immunological dysfunction and emotional and psychological perturbation could indeed provide significant predictive factors for the biologically heterogeneous elements influencing morbidity. This could allow for early intervention with counseling services and relaxation techniques, and therefore offer both a better quality of life and prevent increased morbidity in the immediate and long-term. However, before certainty can replace the "coulds," "mays," and "shoulds," morbidity and mortality associations with emotional states must be better understood, and the efficacy of management of patients found to be in a high risk category proven.

Acknowledgments

In alphabetical order: Dr. Michael Adena, Sue Bartrop-Schneider, Dr. June Crawford, Leesa Croucher, Emeritus Professor Leslie Kiloh, Dr. Rosie Kubb, Dr. Leslie Lazarus,

Elizabeth Luckhurst, Diane Mahoney, Professor David Nelson, Dr. Peggy Nelson, Dr. Don Porritt, Professor Christopher Tennant, Dr. John Wells.
Dr. Roger Bartrop was originally supported by a Research Fellowship from the New South Wales Institute of Psychiatry (1975-1977).
With regard to the longitudinal study, Dr. Bartrop gratefully acknowledges financial assistance from the Staff Specialist Trust Fund and Research Trust Funds and the Department of Radiotherapy at Royal North Shore Hospital (RNSH), Sydney, the New South Wales Institute of Psychiatry, Sydney, and the Department of Psychiatry, Royal Prince Alfred Hospital, Sydney.

CRC Press, Boca Raton, Florida, kindly granted permission to use Table 5 and adjacent text.

Reference Note

Weiner, H. *What the future holds for psychosomatic medicine.* Address to the plenary session of the VII World Congress of the International College of Psychosomatic Medicine, Hamburg (FRG), July 18, 1983.

References

Australian Government Publishing Service. Australian veterans health studies. Commonwealth Institute of Health, University of Sydney, Canberra, 1984.
Bahnson, C. B. Stress and cancer: the state of the art. *Psychosomatics,* 1981, *22,* 207-220.
Baker, R. J., & Nelder, J. A. *The GLIM system-release,* Oxford: Numerical Algorithms Group, 1978.
Bartrop, R. W., Luckhurst, E., Lazarus, L., Kiloh, L. G. and Penny, R. Depressed lymphocyte function after bereavement. *Lancet,* 1977, *1,* 834-836.
Bartrop, R. W., & Porritt, D. W. The biological sequelae of adverse experiences. In A. S. Henderson, & G. D. Burrows (Eds.), *Handbook of social psychiatry.* Amsterdam:

Elsevier, 1988.

Bartrop, R.W., Forcier, L., Jones, M., Kubb, R., Luckhurst, E. & Penny, R. In A.J. Husband (Ed.), *Behaviour and Immunity*. Boca Raton: CRC Press, 1992.

Bartrop, R.W., Craig, A.R., Hancock, K. & Porritt, D.W. Psychological toxicity of bereavement: six months after the event. *Australian Psychologist* (in press).

Breslow, N. E., Lubin, J. H., Marek, P., & Langholz, B. Multiplicative models and cohort analysis. *Journal of the American Statistical Association*, 1983, *78*, 1-12.

Congalton, A. A. *Status and prestige in Australia*. Melbourne: Cheshire, 1969.

Cooper, D. A., Petts, V., Luckhurst, E., Biggs, J. C., & Penny, R. T and B cell population in blood and lymphnode in lymphoproliferative disease. *British Journal of Cancer*, 1975, *31*, 550-558.

Cooperband, S. R. Alpha-globulins affecting the immune response. *Progress in Immunology*, 1974, *2*, 383-389.

Cox, P. R., & Ford, J. R. The mortality of widows shortly after widowhood. *Lancet*, 1964, *1*, 163-164.

Dean, C. & Surtees, P.G. Do psychological factors predict survival in breast cancer? *Journal of Psychsomatic Research*, 1989, *33*, 561-569.

Dixon, W. J., Brown, M. B., Engelman, L. & Jennerich, R. T., & Toporek, J. D. *BMDP statistical software manual*, Vols 1 & 2. 1990. Berkeley: University of California Press, 1990.

Foad, B. S. I., Adams, L. E., Yamauchi, Y., & Litwin, A. Phytomitogen responses of peripheral blood lymphocytes in young and older subjects. *Clinical & Experimental Immunology*, 1974, *17*, 657-664.

Glaser, R., Rice, J., Speicher, C. E., Stout, J. C., & Kiecolt-Glaser, J. K. Stress depresses interferon production by leucocytes concomitant with a decrease in natural killer cell activity. *Behavioural Neuroscience*, 1986, *100*, 675-678.

Greer, S., & Morris, T. Psychological attributes of women who develop breast cancer: a controlled study. *Journal of Psychosomatic Research*, 1975, *19*, 147-153.

Greer, S., & Watson, M. Towards a psychobiological model of cancer: psychological considerations. *Social Science and Medicine*, 1985, *20*, 773-777.

Hamilton, M. A rating scale for depression. *Journal of Neurology, Neurosurgery and Psychiatry*, 1960, *23*, 56-62.

Helsing, K. J., Szklo, M., & Comstock, G. W. Factors associated with mortality after widowhood. *American Journal of Public Health*, 1981, *71*, 802-809.

Irwin, M., Patterson, T., Smith T.L., Caldwell, C., Brown, S.A., Gillin, J.C. & Grant, I. Reduction of immune function in life stress and depression. *Biological Psychiatry*, 1990, *27*, 22-30.

Jackson, D. N. *Personality research form manual.* Goshen, NY: Research Psychologists Press, 1967.

Kiecolt-Glaser, J. K., Garner, W., Speicher, C. E., Penn, G. M., Holliday, J., & Glaser, R. Psychosocial modifiers of immunocompetence in medical students. *Psychosomatic Medicine*, 1984, *46*, 7-14.

Kiecolt-Glaser, J. K., & Glaser, R. Psychological influences on immunity. *Psychosomatics*, 1986, *27*, 621-624.

Kiecolt-Glaser, J. K., Glaser, R., Strain, E. C., Stout, J. C., Tarr, K. L., Holliday, J. R., & Speicher, C. E. Modulation of cellular immunity in medical students. *Journal of Behavioural Medicine*, 1986, *9*, 5-21.

Kronfol, Z., Daniel House, J., Silva Jr., J., Greden, J., & Carroll, B. J. Depression, urinary free cortisol excretion and lymphocyte function. *British Journal of Psychiatry*, 1986, *148*, 70-73.

Levy, S. M., Herberman, R. B., Maluish, A. M., Schlien, B., & Lippmann, M. Prognostic risk assessment in primary breast cancer by behavioural and immunological parameters. *Health Psychology*, 1985, *4*, 99-113.

Linn, B. S., Linn, M. W., & Jenson, J. Anxiety and immune responsiveness. *Psychological Reports*, 1981, *49*, 969-970.

Lynch, J. J. *The broken heart. The medical consequences of loneliness.* Sydney: Harper & Row, 1979.

McNeil, D.R. & Lunn, D. *SPIDA User's Manual.* Sydney: Southwood Press, 1988.

Maddox, J. Psychoimmunology before its time. In News and Views. *Nature,* 1984, 309.

Mason, J. W. Organisation of psychoendocrine mechanisms. A review and reconsideration of research. In N. S. Greenfield & R. A. Sternbach (Eds.), *Handbook of psychophysiology.* New York: Holt, Rinehart & Winston Inc., 1972.

Mechanic, D. The experience and reporting of common physical complaints. *Journal of Health and Behaviour,* 1980, *21,* 146-155.

Nelson, M. Automated screening test for high titre tetanus antibody in donor plasma. *Vox Sang,* 1973, *25,* 457-460.

O'Donnell, M. Endogenous opiates, natural killer cells and psychological factors in early breast cancer patients. In A.J. Husband (Ed.), *Behaviour and Immunity.* Boca Raton: CRC Press, 1992.

Pettingale, K. W., Greer, S., & Tee, D. E. H. Serum IgA and emotional expression in breast cancer patients. *Journal of Psychosomatic Research,* 1971, *21,* 395-399.

Pettingale, K. W. Towards a psychophysiological model of cancer: biological considerations. *Social Science and Medicine,* 1985, *20,* 779-787.

Porritt, D., & Bartrop, R. W. The independence of pleasant and unpleasant affect: the effects of bereavement. *Australian Journal of Psychology,* 1985, *37,* 205-213.

Radloff, L. S. The CES-D scale: a self-report depression scale for research in the general population. *Applied Psychological Measurements,* 1977, *3,* 385-401.

Scherg, H., Cramer, I., & Blohmke, M. Psychosocial factors and breast cancer: a critical evaluation of established hypotheses. *Cancer Detection and Prevention,* 1981, *4,* 165-171.

Schleifer, S. J., Keller, S. E., Camerino, M., Thornton, J. C., & Stein, M. Suppression of lymphocyte stimulation following bereavement. *Journal of the American Medical Association,* 1983, *250,* 374-377.

Schleifer, S. J., Keller, S. E., Myerson, A. T., Raskin, M. J., Davis, K. L., & Stein, M. Lymphocyte function in major depressive disorder. *Archives of General Psychiatry,* 1984, *41,* 484-486.

Schleifer, S. J., Keller, S. E., Siris, S. G., Davis, K. L., & Stein, M. Depression and immunity. Lymphocyte function in ambulatory depressed patients, hospitalised schizophrenic patients and patients hospitalised for herniorraphy. *Archives of General Psychiatry*, 1985, *42*, 129-133.

Sheil, A.G.R. Cancer in dialysis and transplant patients. In P. Morris (Ed.), *Kidney transplantation: principles and practice*. London: Butterworths, 1987.

Siegal, S. *Non-parametic statistics for the behavioural sciences*. New York: McGraw Hill, 1956.

Spielberger, C. D., Gorsuch, R. L., & Lushene, R. E. *Manual for the State Trait Anxiety Inventory*. Palo Alto, CA: Consulting Psychologists Press, 1970.

Templer, D.I. The construction and validation of a death anxiety scale. *Journal of General Psychology*, 1970, *82*, 165-177.

Tennant, C., & Andrews, G. A scale to measure the stress of life events. *Australian and New Zealand Journal of Psychiatry*, 1976, *10*, 27-32.

Watson, M. & Greer, S. Development of questionaire measure of emotional control. *Journal of Psychosomatic Research*, 1983, *27*, 299-305.

Wirsching, M., Stierlin, H., Hoffman, F., Weber, G., & Wirsching, B. Psychological identification of breast cancer before biopsy. *Journal of Psychosomatic Research*, 1982, *26*, 1-10.

World Health Organisation. *Manual of the International Statistical Classification of Diseases, Injuries and Causes of Death* (1975 revision), 1 & 2, 1977.

Young, M., Benjamin, B., & Wallis, C. The mortality of widowers. *Lancet*, 1963, *2*, 454-456.

Ziegler, J. B., Hansen, P., & Penny, R. Intrinsic lymphocyte defect in Hodgkins disease: analysis of the phytohemagglutinin dose-response. *Clinical Immunology and Immunopathology*, 1975, *3*, 451-460.

12

Doctor-Patient Interaction During Daily Ward Rounds: The Traditional Setting and Exploration of the Psychosomatic Approach

Dirk Fehlenberg, Karl Köhle

From the clinical standpoint, the doctor's daily routine ward round has to fulfill several distinct functions. These may be divided into two major groups: the functions which can be related to the management and the organization of the clinical work on the one hand, and the patient-related functions on the other.

Within the group of the managerial and organizational functions three have to be mentioned in particular: (a) the medical council, i.e., the medical discussion of the case concerning the diagnosis, the diagnostics and the therapy, (b) the exchange of information between physicians and the nursing staff and the assignment of diagnostic and therapeutic actions, (c) the supervisory and educational function in relation to medical assistants or students.

The patient-related functions (with primarily physically ill patients) cover at least two points: (d) the (physical) examination including inspection and exploration to make the diagnosis (selective diagnosis), (e) the supervision of the treatment effects. As an active compliance of the patient is generally essential to insure diagnostic and therapeutic steps, there is beside the two aforementioned somatic tasks a further person-related task in the doctor-patient interaction, (f) the task of informing the patient in order to secure his active compliance.

With respect to a biologistic conception of illness and treatment, this person-related task has no value of its own. It is only needed insofar as it helps to secure the somatic functions of the medical treatment. These tasks have to be accomplished basically by two means of interaction: the verbal communication and the physical examination (such as palpation, auscultation, inspection of x-rays, etc.). To take into account the heterogeneity of the clinical functions, it follows that one cannot talk of "the" discourse during rounds. There are several distinct discourses or lines of communication with different groups of speakers and addressees.

The organizational tasks have to be transacted in doctor-doctor, doctor-nurse, or in doctor-assistant communications. The doctor-patient communication itself has a double nature: It has to accomplish the somatic purposes of medical information gathering (for example gathering information about complaints, about the effects and the tolerance of the therapy, etc.) as well as the person-related function of giving medical information to the patient.

This multitude of clinical functions must be remembered if one looks at the patients' point of view. The regular round normally is the only opportunity for the patient to get into contact with the attending doctor. Various medical sociological investigations have shown that hospital patients have strong and partly very specific needs for information (Raspe, 1983). From the patients' point of view, the ward round, especially the doctor-patient talk during the round, should be the institutionalized chance to address their questions to the doctor. The patients therefore should try to intensify the communication with the doctor and particularly the communication about the information they want. So the topic of major importance to the patient is the topic of least importance from the professional standpoint. It is obvious, that a general conflict of interest results between the routine transactions of the staff on the one side and the patients' expectancies on the other side. This general conflict between the expectancies and actions of doctor and patient respectively, has often been described in medical sociology (Reader, Pratt & Mudd, 1957; Friedson, 1961; Waitzkin & Stoeckle, 1972; Siegrist, 1972).

We would like to give a brief summary of some characteristic findings of empirical investigations concerning the interaction during rounds. These findings will show how the above described conflict may be resolved. These findings stem from several investigations carried out at regular rounds in different German hospitals.

First, we will describe a rough characterization of quantitative distribution of some communicative parameters: (a) Although it has to serve various purposes, an average staff-patient contact during the round takes no longer than 3-5 minutes including direct doctor-patient interaction as well as the inside staff talk. (b) The fact that the ward's physician is the only speaker who is actively involved in each communicative line of the round, is reflected by the proportions of utterances contributed by the different speakers: about 50-60% by the doctors, nearly 30% are those of the patient, the rest being contributed by the members of the staff. (c) Only about one fifth of the patients' utterances are initiative, i.e., are not direct reactions to doctors' initiatives (Raspe, 1983). (d) Another investigation has revealed an equal proportion concerning the activity of asking questions: about 80% are the doctors. He uses particular types of questions, which reduce the choice of possible answers. In a typical doctor-patient contact there are between 6 and 11 questions asked by the doctor, but only one by the patient (Nordmeyer, Steinmann, Deneke & Kerekjarto, 1979, 1981; Jährig & Koch, 1982). (e) How do the patients receive the information about their disease? A content analytic study has shown that the patient has to pick up more than 40% of the information, which is relevant to him from the doctor-staff communication. Further on, the information, which the doctor gives in direct communication, is furnished on patients' requests in only one-third compared to two-thirds of all cases, where the doctor gives self-dependent information (Begemann-Deppe, Note 1). (f) This non-consideration seems to be particularly marked when a patient with an unfavorable prognosis is concerned. A by now nearly classical study in the field of German medical sociology done by J. Siegrist (1978) has revealed that doctors reacted to the questions of slightly ill patients in an evasive or incoherent manner 40% of the time, but they did so in more than 90% of the interaction with seriously ill patients. The interpretation for this finding provided by the author is the following: As the seriously ill patient is existentially concerned with his disease in an extreme way, one may conclude that he has comparable high needs for information and social support. As the physicians think along these lines, they act on routine in a particularly rigid and distancing manner.

In conclusion, the aforementioned reported results show that the practical solution for the conflict between the medical routine schedule and the patients' expectancies is that of a non or minimum consideration of the patients' interests.

Following the quantitative investigations some conversation analytic studies have attempted to clear up the question, in what manner and by which communicative means the described asymmetry is produced by the participants in the course of interaction. We will not point out all details that have been described, but we will try to summarize some essential results, that will give a sharpened impression of the central interactional problem of the ward round situation.

What the medical sociologists mean, when they speak of the "asymmetry" of the round (Siegrist, 1978; Raspe, 1983) can be derived from three phenomena. The first is that there are sections in the discourse where the patient is completely excluded from an active participation. The second is that in other phases the patient can participate only as an addressee or as a speaker in a reactive position. And the third is that there are very few initiatives taken by the patient and they are often ignored by the staff.

With respect to the first point, the patients' absolute exclusion from the discourse, can be explained by certain communicative properties of the ongoing discourse within the medical staff. For example, the members of staff speak with low voices, they often use technical terms, abbreviations or elliptic forms of jargon, so that the patient is unable to grasp the objects of reference and/or the topical progression. Further, the talk among the staff is interspersed with completions, clarification requests, corrections, etc., which are transacted rapidly and hinder the patient to see an occasion for getting the floor (Nothdurft, W., 1981; Gück, Matt & Weingarten, Note 4).

In conclusion, there is strong evidence that the communicative inactivity of the patient is at least partly an interactively produced phenomenon. Certain qualities of the doctor-team communication hinder the patients to make their contributions without violating commonly accepted communication postulates as to be relevant, or not to interrupt someone, etc.

The same conclusion may be drawn for the second group of asymmetries. Obviously there are certain communicative strategies of the staff, especially of the doctors, which prevent the patients from taking initiatives, although they are actively taking part in the ongoing discourse as an addressee or as a speaker for answering questions. Here are two examples of this phenomena. First, the physician closes a long explanation addressed to the patient with a question concerning another topic, which has to be answered first. Thereby it becomes impossible for the patient himself to put a question concerning the doctor's explanation (Quasthoff, 1982).

Second, patients are often asked questions which concern topics like their complaints, their sensations, etc., i.e., typical "patients' events" (Labov & Fanshel, 1977). Two phenomena are characteristic of those question-answer sequences: One is that they aim at an information which serves as an argument in the medical considerations of the team. But the formulation of those questions does not give any hint to the medical context. The second phenomenon is that those sequences have a peculiarly shortened form. The switch of the addressee is usually completely unmarked, i.e., there are no vocative and no appropriate turn taking signals. Normally, there are no reactions to the answer of the patient, no comments and no acknowledgements. The linguistic and interactive form of those sequences prevent the patient from adding thematically appropriate comments. One has to conclude that the staff supposes, and uses, the fact that the patient is a constant listener to the medical discourse within the staff, even if he is not addressed. The authors of the investigation which we referred to (Gück et al., Note 2) summarized this situation in the notion of the "permanent communicative availability" of a ward's patient.

A third aspect of the doctor-patient asymmetries becomes obvious when looking at the reactions to the patients' questions. It is rarely the case that a patient at least does not try to answer a physician's question appropriately, but it is quite typical that a patient's initiative, be it some kind of a question or an attempt to tell a story on some occasions, is nullified by different means. When a patient tries to tell a story, the doctor's behavior is characterized by incongruous reactions. Usually he does not give any evaluations, expansions or stimulating remarks etc. Instead the doctor reacts with clarification requests, minimal reactions and functionally equivalent communications which are designed either to stop the patient's probing or to redefine it into the form of a "report" which is more conforming to the professional purposes (Bliesener, 1980; Quasthoff, 1979; Ehlich, Note 3).

A more frequent type of patient response is the request for disease related information. There, too, the physician's typical strategy of "answering" is that of nullifying the patient's aim by certain reactive routines. One investigation has differentiated twelve local strategies of reaction with rejecting effects (Bliesener, 1982). These strategies are short cut solutions to the conflict between the clinical work schedule and the patients' need for information in favor of the former one. Even though they are seemingly successful at the moment, such solutions bear the danger of an escalation in derived conflicts. In general, the patient does not insist on an answer, but he chooses strategies of communication like "boycotting" by minimal reactions or "extend self-representations" which are motivated by his self-respect calling for a repair on the relationship level

(Bliesener & Siegrist, 1981). In such cases physicians quite often use strategies which can be summarized as "humoring the patients' wishes" (Bliesener et al., 1981), such as "promises," "compensation" and "accounts," but they do not change the situation generally. The patient remains excluded from co-determining the interaction of the round.

In the foregoing section we said that the main problem of the traditional round can be found in the large number of competing tasks, respectively in the coordination of different lines of communication. Taking into account the reported phenomena it becomes clear how this problem is solved in the traditional setting. Obviously the coordination is reached in a hierarchical way and the priorities are graded according to the clinical purposes. The organizational tasks and the doctor-staff communication, especially the discussion of the case (doctor-doctor communication) determines the whole structure of the round. These functions have the highest priority. The doctor-patient communication is initiated according to the necessity of the ongoing doctor-team discussion. The person-related task of giving information to the patient (which ideally should be transacted in direct doctor-patient communication) is taken over to a considerable part by the inside staff communication. There is no systematic place in the round for informing the patient. Time, manner and extent are up to the doctors. The patients' interests have the lowest priority. Especially the reactions to patients' initiatives prove that the person-related doctor-patient communication is only realized to an absolute minimum and that it is only used instrumentally for securing the patients' compliance.

A change of the situation towards a better consideration of the patients' interests can only be brought about by changing the institutional and organizational constraints. Such an experiment has been made on the basis of an integrated psychosomatic approach on an internistic ward of the university hospital at Ulm (Köhle, Simons, Böck & Grauhan, 1980). The clinicians restructured the regular round program in order to attain three goals: (1) Dissemination of clinical functions. The tasks relating to the organizational functions ought to be conducted principally in front of the door of the patient's room. The time at the bedside should be for the doctor-patient interaction exclusively. (2) Communicative symmetry. This refers to the verbal behavior on the part of the physicians which serves to attend to and facilitate the patients' desire to communicate. (3) Psychotherapeutic help. One of the central aims of the round's discourse, derived from the basic theorem of the psychosomatic approach that psychic events determine to some extent every disease (Weiss & English, 1944), was to initiate a change of psychic complaints or critical attitudes by psychotherapeutic verbal interventions.

The effects of this approach concerning the clinical reality are reported extensively (Westphale & Köhle, 1982). To summarize the results briefly here, the dissemination of functions was reached completely. The staff's information exchange and the discussion of the case took place before and after the contact with the patient within a span of about 2.5 minutes. Nevertheless, the time spent with the patient was increased to an average of 6.5 minutes. On the whole, this span of time remained for the direct doctor-patient interaction. This makes clear that the problem of coordination is dropped for the psychosomatic round. The physicians, therefore, can give preference to the patients' need to a further extent without running the risk of neglecting the organizational tasks. Corresponding in the Ulm round there are also fewer evasive and nullifying reactions upon patients' initiatives.

These results reveal that the doctor-patient communication can develop along its own lines, freed from competing organizational functions. On the whole the round has to accomplish solely patient-related tasks. However, according to the psychosomatic program, the patient-related tasks were more complex than in the traditional setting.

The physician ought to pay equal attention to each of the following three aspects: information gain, patients' communicative interests, and the psychotherapeutic intervention.

We will concentrate here on the last two points, the consideration of patients' interest and the psychotherapeutic interventions, because in our opinion it is there that the main problem evolves. We would further presume that problems of this structure occur not only in the special case of the psychosomatic round, but in all fields of doctor-patient interaction, which try to cover physical as well as psychic factors in the professional treatment. The problem is that both person-related tasks, "symmetry" and "psychotherapy," become incompatible under certain circumstances. The doctor cannot satisfy both aims in the discourse.

Not wanting to deduce this incompatibility theoretically, we will demonstrate it in a sketch taken from one of our texts. Some background medical information is that the patient is a 73 year old man. The round takes place in the beginning of his stay in the hospital. The man suffers from paroxysmale tachycardia with a long lasting hypertension, a symptom that is comparably not too serious, judged from the medical standpoint. If one takes into account his medical history, one could say that his disease can be seen as part of a more or less expectable physiological decline due to his old age. "Seriousness of disease" and "prognosis" are therefore judged as comparably favorable by the physicians with regard to the disease under treatment. However, from the patient's point of view one has to modify these statements. Besides an appendectomy 24 years ago, this is the patient's first stay in a hospital after a long time. The patient sleeps a lot and even when he is awake he is very inactive. As this behavior is quite unfavorable under the view of rehabilitation, the doctor evidently judges the inactivity as a problem. He tries to relate the patient's inactivity to his stay in the hospital by the following remarks:

> "I want to ask you once again, ah, is it just here in the hospital that you sleep so much, or was it like that at home too? hm, has it (i.e., the inactivity) perhaps something to do with the hospital?"

Moreover, the doctor admonishes the patient to be more active:

> "I would like you to get up as before. I mean, Mr. N., if you are not having a heart attack, you can strain your

heart normally, as you did before. You should have no fear."

It is evident that the physician sees the following connection: The strain of staying in the hospital makes the patient feel depressed. The patient's inactivity is the reaction to his psychic situation and in turn it reinforces the patient's feeling of weakness, etc. The patient, however, interprets the weakness and weariness as the threatening cause. Because he feels weary and exhausted, he behaves, in his opinion, in a cautious way.

Both standpoints remained undiscussed in the first part of the interaction. In the second part the doctor gives some explanations concerning the patient's medication. Subsequently there are the following sequences:

1	Dr.:	mhm
2		Mhm, mhm, is there anything else we can talk about?
3	Pt.:	Well, I don't really know that there is anything.
4	Dr.:	Bye
5	Pt.:	Because they, just what are you going to do so
6		that I may gradually regain my strength. I mean,
7		so that I may be somewhat surer walking?
8	Dr.:	Aha!
9		you mean you can't walk on your own and you still
10		need some sort of assistance?
11	Pt.:	Well, I can walk, but only carefully of course,
12		and only in such a way that I can quickly hold on
13		somewhere.
14	Dr.:	And was it like that before your stay in the
15		hospital?

16	Pt.:	No, no it wasn't like that. Just now.
17	Dr.:	Mhm.
18	Pt.:	because of the treatment.
19	Dr.:	Because of the treatment?
20	Pt.:	Well, mhm, actually as a result of lying in a
21		hospital bed.
22	Dr.:	Mhm.
23	Pt.:	this weakness.
24	Dr.:	Mhm.
25		we'll get our physiotherapist to come and see
26		you and get her to exercise you.
27	Pt.:	Yes.
28	Dr.:	but, it's still quite remarkable that you
29		obviously feel so weakened here in the hospital
30		and after treatment, that you hardly dare get out
31		of bed anymore.
32	Pt.:	Well, I do dare.
33	Dr.:	Mhm.
34	Pt.:	Only I'm simply careful.

Discussion

With the utterance in line 2 the physician explicitly assures the right of the patient to initiate a new topic in the discourse, the latter being limited only to the extent of the most general situational constraints. It is only restricted by the most general situational constraints. The physicians of the Ulm ward have frequently used openers of this kind in order to secure or to allow for a sufficient consideration of the patient's interests. The type used in the text is the most open alternative compared to its functionally equivalent alternatives like: "Do you have any question (left)?" "Anything else, you have on your mind?" or "Anything else I/we can do for you?" etc.

In line 4 it becomes obvious what normally happened if the

patient didn't want to seize the opportunity; i.e., the doctor would initiate the closing. In our text this sequence is stopped, because the patient supplies a response in lines 5-7. Sequences of this kind "firstly a rejection but then the use of an offer" are common phenomena in our texts, that should be analyzed in detail. In our case we presume that it has no substantial effect upon the following turns. We will disregard it, therefore, and concentrate on the patient's comments in lines 5-7 and the subsequent sequences. With regard to its formal speech-act properties, the patient's initiative can be qualified as a question directed to the doctor. The patient wants to know which steps the physician has scheduled for invigorating him. In the context under consideration, this "question" serves as a request for planning and arranging such steps, because it has not been previously discussed that such steps have to be considered. The doctor is particularly obliged to respond to the patient's request, since he himself was responsible for promoting the patient's active participation. He has to suggest a corresponding medical treatment and has to promise its application or otherwise to explain, why such a procedure will be inefficient from the medical standpoint. It is exactly the first alternative that is realized in lines 25-26, i.e., with a delay of 6 turns.

To term this a "delay" is appropriate, because the sequences in lines 8-24 are in no sense necessary steps for answering the patient's demands. In lines 8-10, the doctor explains some presuppositions and the action implied by the patient's question. To demand a professional action, presupposes that the patient thinks he cannot reach an improvement by his own activities. The patient expresses a need for professional help, "what are you going to do . . .," which is interpreted by the physician as a plea for "assistance." As such, the doctor emphasizes the self-responsibility of the patient. These exchanges are in no way necessary for a definite answer to the patient's question. Obviously the physician's utterances aim at another goal than to answer the patient's demand.

The format (i.e., the type of continuity, the formulation, and the intonation) fits the typical format of therapists' utterances in verbal-psychotherapy, e.g. psychoanalysis or Rogerian client-centered therapy. But the patient's response in lines 11-13 doesn't fit the corresponding type of a client's answer. The patient supports his former question by arguing. Obviously he heard the doctor's utterances as a critique, as a critical request for a justification of his proposal. The doctor's question in lines 14-15 are also not essential to assign therapeutical steps. On an earlier occasion in the conversation, the patient had already answered that his weakness and weariness had occurred only since the disease and the therapy. So it is highly probable that the doctor anticipates the patient's negative answer and thereby tries to direct the patient's attention to this "remarkable point" as he formulates it in lines 28-31.

In conclusion it seems to us that in lines 8-24, the doctor tries to draw the patient into a reflecting discourse about the patient's fears, his passivity, and his extreme need for support. This attempt to establish a therapeutically reflecting discourse is interrupted in lines 25-26 with the response actually expected by the patient and then continued in a more explicit way in lines 28-31.

We do not attempt to discuss the doctor's particular techniques nor his actual psychotherapeutic intentions in detail here. What matters for our argument here is the general structure of the problem of action that can be found in the discussed sequence. The notion of "psychotherapy" on the ward round means the correction of disease-related cognitions (emotions, values, elements of knowledge) which don't fit reality. The doctor is in a dilemna as to whenever the patient's cognitions, which prove to be unfounded from the doctor's point of view, lead to a real request for some medical actions (like giving information, a prognosis, or a treatment). The tool of psychotherapeutic intervention is the empathetic and non-appreciative but critical reflecting dialogue which is characterized by a modification, namely a suspension of the well-established form of cooperation that is characteristic for the "everyday discourse" (Flader & Grodzicki, 1982; Koerfer & Neumann, 1982; Ehlich, Note 2).

In a psychotherapeutic setting the therapist generally does

not respond to questions, i.e., he will not give answers but verbalize the cognitions, emotions, values, etc., that are associated with the patient's speech act. If the doctor acts similarly on the round, he obviously offends against the aim of "symmetry." Moreover, as the round is not a psychotherapeutic situation with regard to the expectations of primarily physically-ill patients, the doctor runs the risk of frustrating the patient's attitude of cooperation. He may not be able to reveal the therapeutic purpose (i.e., to establish a mutually defined second order cooperation).

Such feelings of frustration, especially in the beginning of therapy, can also be observed in clients of regular psychotherapy. But clients of psychotherapy can cope more easily with the situation. Certain rites of initiation (as the "basic rule" in psychoanalysis, or the explanation of the procedure in the beginning of Rogerian therapy) as well as the constancy with which the everyday cooperation is withheld, provoke a comparable quick modification of the client's expectation. He learns to prefer the benefits of a long-term therapeutic improvement to the local benefits of getting through his direct communicative interests.

Besides a psychotherapeutic cooperation, the ward requests an everyday form of communicative cooperation in the first place. Compared to regular psychotherapy, this unmodified cooperation does not only concern the preservation of the communication (i.e., the "working relation"), but it concerns real interests of physical treatment. The general problem of a psychosomatically oriented doctor-patient interaction is the necessary switch between two types of discourses which tend to have antagonistic patterns of cooperation. This task can only be solved interactively by a mutual redefinition of the communicative situation. The "good" solution is the participants' mutual agreement with respect to their communicative "frame." So one has to redefine the clinical postulate of "symmetry": The physician should try to facilitate a reciprocity on a meta-level; he should try to facilitate a mutually agreed definition of relationship and of the interactional frames.

The type of communication analysis discussed in this

paper may further a differentiated view of professional problems in psychosomatic doctor-patient interactions and may help to improve the clinical practice. Let us look again at our vignette. We chose this sketch because the doctor's strategy of a relatively short and abrupt switch of cooperative patterns shows concisely the underlying problem. At the same time we have the feeling (we say deliberately "feeling" because up to now we haven't enough safe knowledge about alternatives and their effects) that the procedure chosen by the doctor is an especially risky and problematic one.

In the doctor's utterances, both patterns, the psychotherapeutic and the common pattern of cooperation, are extremely interwoven. This procedure leads to the fact that the switch of the patterns remains unintelligible for the patient. As utterances, which are identical on the surface may have different communicative and interactive implications depending on the specific frame of interaction (i.e. for example different obligations, different potentials with respect to continuity) the patient has to misunderstand the doctor's intention if his interpretation of the frame is different from the doctor's. Let us take, for example, the doctor's turn in lines 9-10. With regard to the common pattern of communicative cooperation, his turn is heard as a request for confirmation. The patient seems to see it that way and reacts with an argumentation that supports his initial question. In a therapeutic frame of reference the doctor's remarks would serve as a verbal therapeutic tool which will normally initiate sequences of negotiation about the aspects of the patient's problem, which are focused in the doctor's utterance (Kindt, 1984). If the patient's reactions don't fit this pattern, there might be two possible interpretations. The patient is either not willing to accept the therapeutic pattern or the patient simply does not see the therapeutic purpose. As in the round, the therapeutic cooperation is not a mutually preestablished pattern—no communication analysis can clear up this point unambiguously. But in our case there is strong evidence that it might be certain features of the doctor's behavior that prevent the patient from seeing the doctor's intention at all.

This analysis remains tentative as long as it cannot be confirmed by the analysis of equally structured passages. Such a systematic communication analysis which starts with the problems of the professionals, but treats them with an independent methodology, would accomplish two functions. First, it will clear up typical types of "misunderstandings" and their possible interactional nature. Thereby it will serve the critical reflection of the professional action independent from the clinical theories. Second, it will work out the comparably favorable alternatives with regard to the handling of the interactive problems.

By use of the term "favorable alternatives" we do not mean a particular fixed communicative strategy, which may be used independently from personal and institutional constraints. In our opinion, this cannot be the aim of a communication analysis. Instead, it could reveal the communicative conditions under which a psychosomatic dialogue can take place and will be acceptable for the patient. In detail, these might be very different proceedings. One of our results is that the physicians of our study showed highly significant inter-individual differences concerning their styles of intervention. They highly differed in their overall number of interventions and showed inter-individual differences in reacting to seriously ill patients. These quantitative differences let us expect a high qualitative variance, too. This variability should help us to find out a variety of ways to manage the problem. These patterns should not serve as fixed routines, but they should be of some help as possible models in the training of interested physicians and medical students.

Reference Notes

1. Begemann-Deppe, M. *Sprechverhalten und Thematisierung von Krankheitsinformation im Rahmen von Stationsvisiten.* Phil. dissertation, Universität Freiburg, 1978.
2. Ehlich, K. *Zur Struktur der psychoanalytischen Deutung.* Unveröffentlicher Aufsatz; Universität Tilburg, 1981.

3. Ehlich, K. *Diskursanalyse von Sprechstundengesprächen*. Vortrag im Kolloquium des SFB 129, Ulm, 1982 (unpublished).
4. Gück, J., Matt, E., & Weingarten, E. *Zur interaktiven Ausgestaltung der Arzt-Patient Beziehung in der Visite*. Manuskript, Institut für Soziale Medizin, FU Berlin, 1983 (to appear in U. Gerhardt et al. [Hg.], Jahrbuch der Medizinsoziologie II. Campus, 1983).

References

Bliesener, T. Erzählen unerwünscht. Erzählversuche von Patienten in der Visite. In K. Ehlich (Ed.), Erzählen im Alltagg, Frankfurt a. M.: Suhrkamp (STW), 1980.

Bliesener, T. *Die Visite—ein verhinderter Dialog*. Initiativen von Patienten und Abweisungen durch das Personal. Tübingen: *Narr*, 1982.

Bliesener, T., & Siegrist, J. Greasing the wheels. *Journal of Pragmatics*, 1981, *5*, 181-204.

Flader, D., & Grodzicki, W. D. Die psychoanalytisch Deutung— eine diskursanalytische Fallstudie. In D. Flader, W. D. Grodzicki, & K. Schröter (Hg.), *Psychoanalyse als Gespräch*. Frankfurt a. M.: Suhrkamp (STW), 1982.

Friedson, E. *Patients view of medical practice*. New York: Russel Sage, 1961.

Franck, D. *Grammatik und Konversation*. Königstein/Ts.: Scriptor, 1980.

Gück, J., Matt, E., & Weingarten, E. Zur alltagssprachlichen Repräsentation intensivemedizinischer Behandlungsroutinen. Zwischenbericht zum Forschungsvorhaben "*Die sprachliche Herstellung und Aufrechterhaltung von Normalitæt in intensivmedizinischen Extremsituationen.*" FU Berlin, *Fachbereich Medizin*, Grundlagenfächer, 1981.

Jährig, C., & Koch, U. Die Arzt-Patient-Interaktion in der internistischen Visite eines Akutkrankenhauses—Eine empirische Untersuchung. In K. Köhle, & H. H. Raspe (Hg.), Das Gespräch während der ärztlichen Visite. München: Urban u. Schwarzenberg, 1982.

Kindt, W. Zur interaktiven Behandlung von Deutungen in Therapiegespræchen. *Journal of Pragmatics*, 1984, *8*, 731-751.

Köhle, K., & Raspe, H. H. (Hg.), *Das Gesprach wæhrend der ærztlichen Visite.* Muenchen: Urban u. Schwarzenberg, 1982.

Köhle, K., Simons, C., Böck, D., & Grauhan, A. (Hg.), Angewandte Psychosomatik. *Die internistisch-psychosomatische Krankenstation—Ein Werkstattbericht.* Basel: Rocom, 1980 (2).

Koerfer, A., & Neumann, C. Alltagsdiskurs und psychoanalytischer Diskurs. In D. Flader, W. D. Grodzicki, & K. Schro er (Hg.), *Psychoanalyse als Gespræch.* Frankfurt a. M.: Suhrkamp (STW), 1982.

Labov, W., & Fanshel, D. *Therapeutic discourse: psychotherapy as conversation.* New York: Academic Press, 1977.

Nordmeyer, J., Nordmeyer, J. P., Deneke, F. W., & Kerekjarto, M. v. Formal—quantitative aspekte des Sprachverhaltens von Arzt und Patient wæhrend der Visite. *Zeitschrift fur Klinische Psychologie*, 1981, *10*, 220-231.

Nordmeyer, J., Steinmann, G., Deneke, F., & Kerekjarto, M. v. Dimensionen des ærztlichen Visitenverhaltens und ihr Zusammenhang mit ausgewæhlten Merkmalen von Arzt und Patient. *Medizinische Psychologie*, 1979, *5*, 208-228.

Nothdurft, W. "Ich komme nicht zu Wort." Austausch-Eigenschaften als Ausschluss -Mechanismen des Patienten in Krankenhaus-Visiten. In W. Frier (Hg.), *Pragmatik/Theorie und Praxis. Amsterdamer Beitræge zur Neueren Germanistik.* Bd. 13. Amsterdam: Rodopi, 1981.

Quasthoff, U. M. Eine interaktive Funktion von Erzæhlungen. In H. G. Soeffner (Hg.), *Interpretative Verfahren in den Sozial—und Textwissenschaften.* Stuttgart: Metzler, 1979.

Quasthoff-Hartmann, U. M. Frageaktivitaten von Patienten in Visitengesprachen: konverstaionstechnische und diskursstrukturelle bedingungen. In K. Köhle, & H. H. Raspe (Hg.), *Das Gœspræch wæhrend der ærztlichen Visite.* Muenchen: Urban u. Schwarzenberg, 1982.

Reader, G. G., Pratt, L., & Mudd, M. C. What patients expect from their doctors. *Modern Hospital*, 1957, *89*, 88-94.

Raspe, H. H. Informationsbeduerfnisse und faktische Informiertheit bei Krankenhauspatienten. In H. Begemann (Hg.), *Patient und Krankenhaus*. Muenchen: Urban u. Schwarzenberg, 1976.

Raspe, H. H. *Information im Krankenhaus*. Gœttingen: Vandenhoeck & Ruprecht, 1983.

Siegrist, J. *Arbeit und Interaktion im Krankenhaus*. Stuttgart: Enke, 1978.

Waitzkin, H. J., & Stoeckle, D. The communication of information about illness. *Advances in Psychosomatic Medicine*, 1972, *8*, 180-215.

Weiss, E., & English, O. S. *Psychosomatic medicine: the clinical application of psychopathology to general medical problems* (reprint). Philadelphia: Saunders, 1944.

Westphale, C., & Köhle, K. Gespræchssituation und Informationsaustausch wæhrend der Visite auf einer internistisch-psychosomatischen Krankenstation. In K. Köhle und H. H. Raspe (Hg.), *Das Gespræch wæhrend der ærztlichen Visite*. Muenchen: Urban u. Schwarzenberg, 1982.

13

Psychosomatic Medicine and Aggression: Theoretical Considerations

Thure von Uexküll

The Problem

Bahnson's identification of a specific psychological syndrome in cancer patients presents from several points of view a challenge to psychosomatic medicine (1964). One of these points of view is expressed in the fundamental question of how medicine can define the concepts "Psyche" and "Soma" in order to be able to relate these processes to each other. Another of these points of view relates to the more specific question: What should our attitude be towards the problem of aggressive drives within the frame of a psychosomatic conceptualization.

One could object that in both cases we are dealing with unnecessary theoretical questions because medicine is an empirical science. Concerning the problem of the relations between theory and empiricism I only wish to say that for me there is no empiricism that does not develop from a theory. It is for this reason that it is essential to reflect on a theory—whatever it may be—in a careful and critical manner. It is for this purpose that the following thoughts attempt to make a contribution. The first part considers the questions raised by a psychosomatic theory or a given psychosomatic model. The second part deals with the question of how to define the problem of aggression within such a theoretical framework.

Considerations Concerning the Problem of a Psychosomatic Theory

The first sketch of a psychosomatic model and a corresponding theory extensive enough to meet the requirements that must be demanded of such concepts, was developed by Freud. One does not find his psychosomatic model in his concept of conversion, but in his drive theory, which he had already conceived in 1895 in his "Entwurf einer Psychologie." In spite of all his later variations, he basically held on to this formulation throughout his life.

At that time Freud wrote that the Psi-System, i.e., the psychological system, was a defenseless target for the endogenous drive potentials, and that the resulting excitations were the driving forces for the psychological mechanisms. Freud states: "What we know about the endogenous excitation potentials can be expressed by the assumption that they are of an intercellular nature, that they arise continuously, and that they only periodically emerge as psychological drives." In this manner a model has been sketched in which an intercellular chemical reaction is transformed into a psychological excitation only periodically, i.e., only under certain conditions. He writes (1895, p. 402): "We know this power as 'will,' the descendent of the drives." (Translation into English by Claus B. Bahnson.) Two points brought out in this formulation are important:

1. The distinction between intercellular processes, that have to be described in concepts belonging to physics and chemistry and, as we would say nowadays, unfold within the organism as a relatively closed system on the one side, and processes in the Psi-System on the other side, for the description of which other concepts become necessary. One of Freud's great contributions is, as we all know, the development of a

language with which it has become possible to describe these experiential phenomena.

2. The observation that transformations between the system of intercellular chemical processes and the Psi-System take place periodically, i.e., that transformations take place only under certain conditions.

In this way two great research themes have been formulated. The first is the epistemological theme of the differences and the relationships between a system of intracellular chemistry and a system of psychological processes. This theme is only now beginning to take on shapes that may allow us to construct concrete models for empirical research. In order to make this possible—and I shall return to this point later—the development of a general systems theory and a general semiotic science were necessary preconditions.

The second important research theme is expressed in a question concerned with the conditions necessary for the realization of interactions between intraorganismic, i.e., somatic processes, and psychological processes. This second theme concerned with the conditions under which intracellular chemical reactions become psychological stimuli, and vice versa, was already being dealt with by Pavlov during Freud's lifetime.

It is necessary to deal with both themes in order to answer the question of how we today can conceptualize a psychosomatic theory and a psychosomatic model. Freud himself did not take part in the further development of these two themes. As he formulated it in a letter to Viktor von Weizsäcker, for didactic reasons he felt that he himself and his associates were committed to concentrate on the great task of developing a language for an empirically demonstrable and therapeutically effective psychology. However, his outline of a psychosomatic theory and the early models have remained the basis for later developments.

Freud's first draft starts out by describing a hypothetical *somato-psychological* process. A concentration of chemical substances in the body is transformed into a psychological drive. In 1895 nobody yet knew about such chemical substances, and Freud probably thought primarily about the sexual chemicals. The concept of hormones was first formulated in 1902 by Bayliss and Starling. However, since Claude Bernard, one had become aware of the concept of the "Milieu interne" and of the general concept of a balance, or interaction between the internal and the external milieu, so that these formulations probably were forerunners of Freud's concept.

The *psychosomatic* aspect of the model is contained in the concept that the psychological drives initiate activities, which (i.e., via sexual satisfaction) then have a cybernetic effect on the intracellular chemistry, and at this site reduce the very source of the psychological drive. With the concept of a somato-psychological drive source and a psychosomatic drive discharge, a sketch of a cybernetic circle with negative feedback—as one would say in our contemporary terminology—had been presented, which integrated two heterogeneous phenomenal areas: a Psi-System encompassing psychological processes and a somatic system involving intercellular chemical reactions (see Figure 1).

**Figure 1
Psi-System**

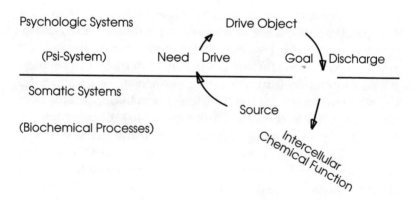

Legend: Freud described in 1915 (in "Triebe und Triebschicksale") four criteria for a drive: The need, the source, the goal, and the object. Among these, the source refers to the intercellular chemical processes resulting in a disturbance of homeostasis, which can be re-established and re-balanced only through the use of compensatory possibilities in the environment (the object of the drive.)

Such a model, however, necessarily remains misty and elusive. In order to develop a tool for empirical research on the basis of such a model, it becomes necessary to clearly formulate the differing natures of the two areas and the problem of their linkage with each other. As already stated, only with the advent of systems theory and the science of semiotics were the possibilities created to initiate these steps. Thus, I shall briefly refer to both of these theoretical developments dealing with epistemological and conceptual themes.

Systems theory has developed a concept of a hierarchically structured order in which repeatedly less complex systems (i.e., cells) are integrated as elements or sub-systems into more complex systems (i.e., organs), which then again serve as elements in even more complex systems (i.e., organisms). Thus, one can continue to distinguish a hierarchy of levels of integration all the way up to social systems in such a way that given levels of integration become the subject matter of specific disciplines, for example, chemistry or biology. The stepwise hierarchies, then, are the subject matters of physics, biology, psychology, and sociology.

Systems theory, through its emphasis on the concept of "integration" and "levels," or "steps" brings into focus a state of affairs that had so far been ignored, although this fact had already been clearly formulated by Ehrenfels, the founder of Gestalt Psychology, during the last century. A whole system is more than the sum of its parts. Formulated in a different way, it means that with the development of a system, new aspects or characteristics appear that do not yet appear on the sub-system levels. This condition has been described as "emergence." The Nobel prize recipient P. B. Medawar (1977) describes this phenomenon in the following way:

> As we go up the hierarchy...we find that the informational content and empirical richness of the sciences progressively increase—as is to be expected—partly because each science contains the theorems of the sciences below it, and partly because the restrictions progressively imposed on possible interactions be-

tween constituent parts bring it about that each higher-level subject contains ideas and conceptions peculiar to itself. These are the "emergent" properties.

For our problem it means the following: With the transition from simpler to more complex system levels, we see that new phenomena appear in sudden leaps. This holds first of all for the transition from a level of inorganic material to a level of biological systems, then again with the transition from biological to psychological systems, and, finally, from the psychological to the social systems levels. These jumps force us, whenever we arrive at the level of a new scientific discipline, to develop a new terminology, i.e., a language that makes it possible to describe the properties and new aspects of the emerging phenomena.

Physics, biology, psychology, and sociology each need new scientific languages in order to describe the phenomena observed on their levels of discourse. Languages cannot easily be translated from one to the other, and most importantly, cannot be reduced to the language of the science on a simpler or subordinate level of organization. This realization helps to clarify the problem of how to conceptualize the relationships among these heterogeneous levels of observation.

Freud's drive model attempts to visualize the connection between the level of biological processes in the body, which may be described on a biochemical level, and the level of psychological processes, which can be understood only through the use of psychological concepts. The systems' theoretical approach thus allows us to define more precisely the different levels of the drive model and to delineate these levels in their relationships to one another. But only the modern semiotics theory gives us an answer to the question of how to conceptualize the connection between the different levels of integration. Semiotics states the necessity for developing new languages to describe phenomena on each new (higher) level of integration, based on the assumption that very specific sign processes exist on each of these levels of organization, which maintain the organization of, and connection among, the elements of the contributing systems belonging to this level.

In this way, as far as we know today, the sign processes of the genetic codes communicate the exchange of information among different cellular elements, on the level of the cell. On the level of the organism, hormones and nervous action potentials carry the transmission of information among the organs; and on the next higher level, the psychological processes are responsible for the transmission of information between the organism and the environment. On each of these levels we encounter a sign system that is specific for this particular level of observation and functioning.

The problem of how the connections among the different levels of the system's hierarchy should be conceptualized had never been recognized previously. The first assumption was that the languages of the different sciences could be reduced to the language of physics. This assumption was the basic dogma of the natural sciences during the nineteenth century. Freud and Pavlov still believed in this dogma, which was only overcome and revised through the development of quantum physics during the twentieth century. From a systems theoretical point of view it is possible to formulate the problem, that becomes visible through the concept of a hierarchical order, as a question about how "upward directed effects" and "downward directed effects" come about within such a hierarchy. Concretely this can be expressed in the question: How can processes that take place within the cell produce "upward directed effects" in organs, organisms and social systems, i.e., in a family; and how, to move the other way, do "downward moving effects" come about, i.e., in the cells of the organism of a member of a family in which particular pathogenic constellations are at play?

The so-called psycho-physiological problem appears only as one of many problems within the frame of such a hierarchical conceptualization. Analogous problems appear at every border between the levels or layers of a hierarchically developed system.

A semiotic theoretical analysis shows that these problems

can be resolved only through a translation from one sign system to another. Freud's assumption concerning a periodical transposition of intercellular chemical reactions into a psychologically experienced need means, within the framework of this conceptualization, that such translations from one level to another come to pass only under certain, periodically returning conditions.

This necessarily only vaguely formulated hypothesis in Freud's draft of a model found an empirical support and operationalization in Pavlov's empirical research. The significance of Pavlov's research for the drive concept and for a new psychosomatic theory has hardly been understood as yet. The process, which Pavlov described as the formation of a conditioned reflex or as conditioning, is nothing less but a translation from a psychological semiotic system into a system of somatic signals, and vice versa. This translation represents a connection between a psychological and a somatic level that does not even exist without this translation.

As we have previously expressed it (von Uexküll and Wesiack, 1979) a "transmission of meaning" takes place in the following way: Signs, that communicate messages within the body concerning the significance of an organ reaction for other organs, are geared to other signs, that inform the organism of processes taking place in his environment, and which now take on significance for the organ reactions.

Pavlov also said that such linkages or translations of meanings come about only "periodically," i.e., only in situations in which certain conditions have been established, and that the duration of such interlocking systems depends on the maintenance of such conditions. In the well-known example Pavlov's research dogs began to excrete stomach juices and saliva in response to the noises produced by the laboratory assistant next door who was preparing the dog food. This secretion had previously started only at the time when taste, smell and tactual stimuli had been translated into nerve signals for the activation of the saliva and stomach glands. Now auditory stimuli, that previously had remained neutral, were locked into the relevant signals in the nervous system. This interlocking of auditory stimuli, that oriented the dogs about events in their environment, with the nervous signals in their bodies, was, however, taking place only when the dogs were both hungry and healthy. When they were sated (full) or sick, conditioning did not take place.

I refer to these old and well-known observations for two reasons:

1. Because they show that the "periodicity" emphasized by Freud can be explained on the basis of an individual readiness, or to put it differently, an organismic openness or vulnerable phase as a precondition for the establishment of such psychophysiological linkages or translations.

2. Because they make explicit that with respect to animals and even more pointedly, in the case of human beings, we must take into account not only those aspects of physiology that appear uniform for all individuals of the class, but also an individual physiology applied to specific organs. The stomach and saliva glands of the Pavlovian dogs developed since the time of their conditioning an individual physiology that differed from the physiology of the stomach and saliva glands of non-conditioned animals. The individual physiology can only be understood on a biographical basis, i.e., only on the basis of knowledge of the individual history, pertaining to those situations in which new linkages of meanings either had taken place or had not taken place.

Pavlov had thus through his research supplied Freud's biographical drive model with a psychosomatic dimension. However, these relationships only become visible when one considers the concepts in the light of systems theory and the theory of semiotics.

Considerations Regarding the Problem of Aggressive Drives

What does the problem of aggressive drives look like within the framework of such a theory? Within such a framework the concepts "somatic" and "psychological" are not only formally defined as designations of different levels of integration with specific sign systems, but are also content-wise endowed with different functions. The concept "somatic" is reserved for semiotic or sign processes that unfold within the organism between cells and organs. The body is defined as a relatively closed system, for the function of which environmental events are nearly irrelevant. The concept "psychological," in contrast, is applied to semiotic processes which inform the organism about events in its environment, i.e., concerning drive objects. The psychological sign processes cut out a section from the environment of the living system, a section that is determined by the existing drives and needs. They build up a subjective "environment" around the living being that can be experienced by this particular living being only, but by no external observer. The psychological semiotic processes, according to a concept developed by Jakob von Uexküll (1920), form a subjective sphere created by the sensory apparatus of the organism as an invisible bubble surrounding the body, invisible to others, which is in a certain sense an extension or additional compartment of the body.

In other words, the concepts "body" and "soul" described two different forms of organization, one of which is designated as plant-like or vegetative. From the point of view of the vegetative system, no environment yet exists subjectively for this "body." This state corresponds to the condition of plants in winter hibernation, of seeds, of bird eggs during hatching or of mammals during the embryonic phase. For the maintenance of life and these conditions, the necessary metabolic processes take place on the basis of reserves that either are built into the organism (i.e., the egg) or, as is the case with mammalian embryos, are delivered and made available by the mother organism. Freud developed the concept of primary narcissism to describe this condition. During this time all drive forces are believed to be directed inward. The organism is in a certain sense its own love object.

The other form of organization of somatic and psychological levels of integration with specific sign systems corresponds to the condition that holds after the end of the embryonic existence, i.e., for mammals after birth, when the reserves are no longer delivered by the mother organism, but must be drawn from the environment by the young organism itself. From this point in time, a construction of the subjective environment through psychological sign processes becomes a precondition for survival. In order to emphasize this point, we talk here about an "animalistic" level of organization in contrast to the vegetative level; thus psyche is called "anima" in Latin (Bateson, 1979).

In a systems theoretical formulation, this means the following: After the stress of birth the organism must jump from the simpler, vegetative level of integration (as "body only") to a more complex level of organization. The organism can now survive only as a system consisting of at least two subsystems, a body and a system built on psychological sign processes relating to the outer world.

This introductory comment is necessary in order to understand why Freud only relatively lately considered the existence of an aggressive drive and why he tried to introduce such a complicated metaphysical construction with his "death drive." Freud started off with the concept of primary narcissism, based on the concept that early psychological development initiates within a vegetative form of organization that functions as a relatively closed system. In this model the libidinous drives reign supremely. An aggressive drive can only be introduced artificially as an afterthought within a sequence of complicated theoretical supportive structures. Even more importantly, the catastrophe for the infant at birth of immediately being confronted with the vital demand of establishing a new level of integration, remains unrecognized. A great deal of the uncertainty that has characterized the discussion of aggressive drives in psychoanalytic theory and has led to new attempts at formulations (Harmann, Kris & Loewenstein, 1949) may have its roots in this lack of awareness of a shift at the time of birth.

In this area change has occurred only with the introduction of the idea that psychological development takes place in a setting of primary social unity that is first introduced by the mother-child symbiosis or dyad. This concept mainly developed in connection with works by Ferenci, by Melanie Klein, M.

Balint, Margaret Mahler, D. W. Winnicott and others, has unlocked a number of other new aspects which are still unsettled. Just the same, the first outlines of a new organization and evaluation have clearly become visible.

Thus, today it is possible to contrast the "physiological drives," serving the maintenance of homeostasis within the organism and thus representing the "egotistic interests" of the body, with the aggressive and sexual drives, which are social in the sense that they aim at the "altruistic goals" of incorporating the organisms within social systems. In contrast to hunger and thirst, that remain "private business," hate and love necessarily demand a social counterpart. Thereby the questions about which functions to ascribe to these drives also change.

However, with this concept we have also reintroduced "respectable methodological and philosophical problems, related to the very origin of psychological activities" (Fornari, 1970). The consequences have been most impressively introduced by Winnicott with his concept of the primary identity of the child and mother (D. W. Winnicott, 1945, 1956, 1958, 1967, 1971). Because important aspects of the significance of aggressive drives for psychosomatic relationships are coming to the fore here, I will try to describe his concept in a very shortened form.

Basically new in Winnicott's contribution is the thesis that in the primary symbiotic unit, mother and child do not exist as two beings, but are identical. This early identity, furthermore, forms the basis for our experience of being, anteceding all experiences of drive. All of this refers to the creation of a supra-subjective and supra-objective unity.

Translating this thesis into our terminology we find that it expresses two aspects:

1. Psychological being, which we have defined as a semiotic process informing the organism about events of vital significance in the environment, grows out of the identity with the first vital and significant environmental event, namely the encounter with the mother.

2. Psychological existence is a new creation, i.e., an expres-

sion of the emergence of new phenomena associated with the formation of a system on a level more complex than the somatic.

Winnicott has thereby created a new definition of the concept "being," a concept with which philosophy has grappled for over two thousand years. His definition differs both from the definition of Descartes, who links the concept of being to thought (cogito ergo sum), as well as from that of Berkeley, for whom being is sensory perception (esse est percipi). For Winnicott, being means existence on the level of psychological integration.

Winnicott (1974) talks about "object relationships" in order to describe the early identity of subject and object. This identity remains the hidden background for our relationships to the world throughout our life span in spite of all the losses and separations in our lives, and the repeated differentiation. In the earliest form of this relationship, the child is the mother, in the same sense that the mother in her affective experience is her own child. From Winnicott's point of view, the criterion of the "sufficiently good mother" is her capacity to experience herself as her own child and to be able to wait for the moment at which the child is able to "create the motherly breast for himself". Interestingly, this concept is closely affiliated with that of J. H. Mead, for whom the formation of the self and of the social development depend on the experience of exchange of roles, in which each partner through adopting the role of the other takes over a bit of the other's identity.

For our discourse, however, the greatest interest centers around the function and role of the aggressive drive within the frame of Winnicott's concepts. This drive enables the child to untie itself from the identity of the mother and to arrive at the first experiences of a self. The earliest willful motoric actions, i.e., the "perception" of the intentions that lead to motoric activities, initiates the dramatic development that begins with the separation from the mother and that finally leads, when everything goes well, to the creation of a self and a world populated with independent objects.

In this way the child destroys the "subjective object," as

Winnicott calls the dyadic mother. Because she, on her part, experiences the child as a part of herself, these efforts on the part of her child to become independent are perceived as a destructive insult. Mother's job is now to survive this "being destroyed" without retaliating upon her child. Only in this way can she give the child the chance to discover the mother as an "objective object" with whom one can interact and thereby experience oneself as an independent being.

That is Winnicott's starting position in a very condensed form. The vicissitudes around the discovery of the "objective object" appear to Winnicott to be—and I can only touch on this briefly here—a very long and dangerous developmental process throughout, that can succeed only via intermediary steps. Among these steps the phase of omnipotence and megalomanic fantasies is of particular importance. Only the certainty that mother can be recreated whenever she is needed gives the child freedom from anxiety necessary to avoid experiencing the deadly danger presented by the destruction not only of the dyadic mother, but also of oneself due to one's increasing independence. I think that an important aspect of aggressiveness is becoming clearly defined here. Every act or activity that pushes beyond the original borders entails omnipotence fantasies, even if they are well defended against or completely hidden.

What are the consequences of this outline for the existence of an aggressive drive and the difference between this drive and other drives? As far as I can see, we are here dealing with two points within the framework of a psychosomatic drive theory, where the one concerns the classification, the other point concerns the function of drive potentials.

1. Regarding the first point, I have already touched upon the possibility that one might consider libidinal and aggressive drive tensions as social drives, in contrast to the so-called physiological drives that are somatically and individually defined.

2. The second point relates to the necessity of re-evaluating the purposes of libidinal and aggressive drive potentials within the framework of the human cultural development. From

Freud's conceptual point of view, aggressive drives are destructive to culture. They block or destroy the formation of social groups and cultural relationships that can exist only on the basis of libidinal drive potentials. According to the concept of the primary dyadic unity the process looks different. Now the libidinous drives extinguish the individuality of the subject. The individuality is again absorbed in a social unit or oneness. This tendency is made quite clear in the sexual drive. However, this tendency can also be observed as a pressure towards conformity in political groups and in the longing to submit to this pressure. We recognize this tendency in the so-called mass-phenomena. The aggressive drive, in sharp contrast to this tendency to fuse, has as a goal to differentiate and delineate the individual as a unit within the social group. This drive is the necessary condition for the structurization of the social group.

Within this context, pain also appears in a new light. Pain, closely associated with aggressiveness, produces the border differentiating the own body from all other objects, that are not part of the self. Those who cause us pain push us back within the borders of our own bodies.

From a genetic point of view, the aggressive drive thus develops as a drive aimed at the self-sufficiency of the own ego. The aggressive drive destroys the primary identity with the object and blocks the re-establishment of this primary identification, that constantly threatens our individuality as libidinal temptation.

Complex and differentiated social units can only be understood as a sophisticated interplay involving both drive forces, always balanced off against each other on new levels of integration and in continually new configurations of tension.

This concept can explain a number of phenomena that otherwise remain puzzling. Within the animal world we can mention, for example, phenomena such as a distance of flight, a pecking order, or defense of "turf." Regarding the development of the aggressive drive in the human, two questions in particular seem to play a decisive role:

1. the degree to which the single person has been able to

separate from the dyadic mother and to develop an individual ego;

2. to which degree has it or has it not become possible to come to terms with his own omnipotent conflictual needs.

What can be said about psychosomatic aspects of aggressiveness within this theoretical frame? I shall restrict myself to a few remarks that may suggest in which way numerous observations can be re-interpreted in a new way within the frame of a system and theoretically oriented socio-psychobiology.

We can then observe that systems on any level of integration show resistance against being incorporated at the next higher and more complex level. Systems on any level of integration develop their quality of a "self" into a specific sign system. Such sign systems can be observed on the different levels of integration. On the biological level the immune system has the task to differentiate between the "self" and "non-self." Sebeok (1979) cites in this relationship R. A. Good who writes:

> The immune reaction has two fundamental components: Recognition and response, or how an antigen— defined as any object that provides an antibody response—is recognized, and how a structure exactly complementary to it is synthesized...The qualifying property of an antigen is its foreigness—its property of being non-self...In brief, the immunological system functions as a prime defense against infection and thus is pivotal in maintenance of body integrity by distinguishing between "self" and "non-self."

With the development of a centralized nervous system the sign system "pain" emerges and takes over a similar task for the total organism. In the human, the specific sign system for "anxiety" is added during a particular developmental phase. Anxiety seems to serve the task to supervise and guard the belongingness to a particular social unit, i.e., to defend this unity as "self" against strangers as "non-self."

Research concerning the effects of early separation of

young animals from their mother animals by Harlow with primates, Henry with mice, and Weiner with rats, demonstrates the overwhelming importance of the symbiotic phase for the linking of meaning between the first environmental stimuli and the somatic sign processes within the body. They suggest that also the linking of the sign processes on the biological, psychological, and social levels of the self can be disturbed irreversibly during this phase, so that an existence as an individual in a social group only becomes possible within the setting of more or less severe restrictions, limitations, and risks.

Many observations speak in favor of the notion that the results of these animal studies may be generalized to humans, and that many observations concerning psychosomatic relationships must be re-interpreted from this point of view. When we attempt such a re-interpretation two particularly important developmental paths seem to emerge as precursors of pathological predispositions.

The first can be described in the following manner: When aggressiveness as a social drive defends our individuality against being absorbed or incorporated in a social system, the following question emerges as paramount: How well or poorly has a human being succeeded in separating from the early identity with the mother and to build a stable self? The person who repeatedly must prove his value both to himself and to others through the satisfaction of his fantasies of omnipotence and having great importance, is living in a reality in which in one moment a triumph can promote the feeling of having a self, only to experience the destruction of the self in the next moment when no triumphs are in sight. The "behavior pattern A" seems to be a variant of this type of developmental pathology.

The other predisposition seems to have to do with the complex of symptoms described by Bahnson. Concerning Bahnson's complex of symptoms an interpretation presents itself, which starts with the following question: What happens when the child destroys the dyadic mother with his early aggressiveness, and when after the destruction of the subjective inner object he remains unable to find or identify the mother as an outer objective object? Winnicott suggests that the "intermediate playful relationship" with the mother then cannot be established, so that the child is deprived of the experience of defining himself in the mirror of the mother. Winnicott, referring also to Lacan, talks about "the mirror function of play." He tells about a female patient, whose central problem was her own identity, that her association to the story concerning "mirror, mirror on the wall," from the fairytale about Snow White, was expressed in the suggestion: "It would be awful, when a child looks into the mirror and sees absolutely nothing!"

Terrible and awesome, because the blind mirror presents the unexplainable indictment of oneself for carrying the guilt for the expulsion from paradise. But it is also doubly horrible, the early identity being so fragile, that no firm feeling of *being* could be established. The child must then later, in addition to suffering from unexplainable guilt feelings, also tolerate living a life in an unreal world, so frequently described by depressive patients. To function in a barren and sad reality presents the constant stress of being weighted down, so that a renewed object loss then may be perceived as the final catastrophe.

Bahnson has summarized the conditions that he has observed in many cancer patients (1964, 1986) after describing the biography of a young patient who died of metastasized breast cancer when she was only twenty-eight:

1. Childhood trauma, loss of love object, lack of parental emotional warmth and protection;

2. Main mood coloring all experiences: The expectancy, or even certainty, that everything must go wrong combined with guilt feelings for these failures;

3. A repetition compulsion involving self-destructive behaviors;

4. The development of a "double life" or a "double self" in which realistic and adaptive ego operations exist parallel to, but separated from underlying existing feelings of being wounded, not to be loved, to be isolated, and of forever being abandoned.

He states that "these overwhelming or traumatic experiences set in motion long-term and chronic disturbances, which destabilize the psycho-biological balance and make the person vulnerable to illness. Combination of the chronic disturbance with later relevant life stress has as a result that the existing and otherwise functional realistic adaptional efforts fail and, due to lack of flexibility, are unsuccessful in warding off the stress."

In the case of these patients, the interpretation presents itself that subsequent to the primary disturbance of the balance between aggressive and libidinal drives, also later in their lives no balance could be established between the destruction of and fusion with the original object. For the cancer patient, no warmth of the internalized mother protects against hardships, and when the weak shell of a fragile external object also is lost later in life, no image is left in the mirror.

In closing I would like to offer for discussion my considerations concerning the following hypothesis: Do we not pursue a phantom when we search for an isolated, independent aggressive drive? Is Freud's early formulation not more realistic than his later concept of eros/thanatos? Originally he held the opinion that the destructive drive only was one form of expression of the sexual drive. When we re-approach these formulations the question then presents itself whether aggression and libido are not in reality two aspects of one and the same force, which mutually determine each other and, in a variety of combinations and interactions, always complement each other—very much as it is the case with electrical currents, where the interaction of negative and positive charges presents a similar picture?

In this case situations would become pathogenic whenever a disbalance occurred in which one polarity would gain preponderance over the other, or when conditions prevailed which would lead to a sudden dislodging of the two interlocked polarities, in case that these would not then be re-combined and reconciliated in a new way and thus be partially neutralized. In the introduction to the famous, or infamous, "Histoire d'O," presenting the history of a masochistic passion, one finds reference to a peculiar report concerning the dangerous effects of such an "unlocking"— or "splitting"—of hate and love in the reality of the social world under the headline: "A revolution on Barbados":

> A peculiar rebellion during the year 1838 resulted in many bloody massacres on the otherwise peaceful island of Barbados. Approximately two-hundred black persons, men and women, all set free by the March decree of release from prison, located and visited one morning their previous master, a certain Glenelg, and asked him to accept them back as his slaves. A written complaint, authored by an anabaptist pastor, was presented and read aloud. Then the discussion began. But Glenelg would not be talked into repossessing his previous slaves due to timidity, uncertainty, or perhaps simply out of anxiety for breaking the law. In response the blacks first tried to gently convince him, but then subsequently massacred him and his whole family. Still on the same evening they returned to their huts where they took up their usual palaver, familiar work and rites. The whole event could quickly be quelled by the interception of Governor MacGregor, and the general liberation continued its progress.

I think that this report conveys an impression of the explosive forces which in a great variety of mixtures of aggression and libido exist as dormant powers on all levels of our lives.

References

Bahnson, C. B., & Bahnson, M. B. Cancer as an alternative to psychosis: a theroetical model of somatic and psychologic regression. In D. M. Kissen & L. L. LeShan (Eds.), *Psychosomatic aspects of neoplastic disease*. Philadelphia, PA: Lippincott, 1964.

Bahnson, C. B. Das krebsproblem in psychosomatischer sicht. In Th. von Uexküll (Hrsg.), *Psychosomatische medizin*. Munchen: Urban & Schwarzenberg, 1986.

Balint, M. *Primary love and psychoanalytic technique.* London: Tavistock Publication, 1965.

Bateson, G. *Geist und nature: eine notwendige einheit.* Frankfurt: Deutsch, 1982.

von Bertalanffy, L. *General system theory.* New York: G. Braziller, 1968.

von Ehrenfels, Ch. *Wörterbuch der Philosophie.* Stuttgart: Schwabe & Co., 1974.

Ferenci, S. *Schriften zur Psychoanalyse.* Frankfurt: Fischer Verlag, 1970.

Fornari, F. *Psychoanalyse des ersten Lebensjahres.* Frankfurt: Fischer Verlag, 1970.

Freud, S. Neu: 1950, Entwurf einer psychologie. In: Aus den Anfangen der psychoanalyse. London: 1895.

Freud, S. *Zur Einführung des Narzismus.* GW. Bd 10, 1914.

Freud, S. *Triebe und triebschicksale.* GW. Bd 10, 1915.

Freud, S. *Jenseits des Lustprinzips.* GW. Bd 13, 1920.

Good, R. A. *Immunology: the many-edged sword.* New York: Braziller, 1974.

Harlow, H. F., & Zimmerman, R. R. Affectional responses in infant monkey. *Science,* 1959, *130,* 141.

Harmann, H., Kris E., & Loewenstein, R. M. Notes on the theory of aggression. *Psychoanalytic study of the child,* 1949, *3/4,* 9.

Henry, J. P., & Stephens, P. M. *Stress, health and the social environment: a sociobiological approach to medicine.* New York: Springer, 1977.

Klein, M. *Das Seelenleben des Kindes und andere Beitrege zur psychoanalyse.* Reinbeck: Rowohlt, 1962.

Mahler, M. S., Pine, F., & Bergmann, A. *Die psychische Geburt des Menschen.* Reinbeck: Rowohlt, 1980.

Medawar, P. B., & Medawar, J. S. *The life science.* New York: Harper & Row, 1977.

Sebeok, Th. A. *The sign and its masters.* Austin, Texas: University of Texas Press, 1979.

von Uexküll, Th., & Wesiack, W. *Lehrbuch der Psychosomati Medizin.* Muenchen: Urban & Schwarzenberg, 1979.

von Uexküll, J. *Theoretische Biologie.* Berlin: Springer, 1920.

von Uexküll, J. *Bedeutungslehre, ambrosius barth.* Leipzig: Springer, 1940.

Weinger, H. *Psychobiology and disease.* New York: Elsevier, 1977.

Winnicott, D. W. *Vom spiel zur realität.* Stuttgart: Klett Verlag, 1971.

Winnicott, D. W. *Playing and reality.* New York: Penguin Books, 1974.

List of Contributors

Bartrop, Roger W., M.D., Clinical Senior Lecturer, University of Sydney; Senior Staff Specialist, Psychiatry, Royal North Shore Hospital, Sydney, Australia

Baumann, Thomas, M.D. Psychosomatic Department, University of Munich, Pittenkofer Strasse 8A, 8000 Munich, Germany

Bilek, Hans-Peter, M.D., Doctor of Psychiatry and Neurology, Vienna, Austria

Boll, Annegret, Ph.D., Clinical Psychologist, Institute of Rehabilitation at Bad Segeberg, Bad Segeberg, West Germany

The late Cousins, Norman, Past Professor, and Chairperson, of the Psychoneuroimmunology Task Force at the School of Medicine, University of California, Los Angeles, California, United States

Dyregrov, Atle, Ph.D., Director, Center for Crisis Psychology, Bergen, Norway

Engelman, Suzanne R., Ph.D., Formerly Assistant Clinical Professor, Department of Psychiatry, University of California, San Francisco Medical School; Private Practice, San Jose, California, United States

Fehlenberg, Dirk, Ph.D., Clinical Psychologist, PLK Weisseman, Ravensburg, Germany

Fleck, Stephen, M.D., Professor Emeritus of Psychiatry and Public Health, Yale University; Supervisor and Consultant, Clinical Services, Department of Psychiatry, Yale University; Supervisor and Consultant, Greater Bridgeport Mental Health Center, New Haven, Connecticut, United States

Forcier, Lina, Ph.D. Institute of Occupational Health and Safety, Quebec, Canada

Hertz, Dan G., M.D., Professor of Psychiatry, Hebrew University—Hadassah Medical School; Director, The Dr. Walter Schindler Center for Medical Psychotherapy, Hadassah University Hospital and Medical Center, Jerusalem, Israel

Jacob, Wolfgang, M.D., Professor Emeritus of Social Medicine, University of Heidelberg, Thomastrasse 30, 8204 Brannenburg, Germany

Jones, Michael, BSc (Hons.), Biostatistician, Health Information Systems Department, Royal North Shore Hospital, Sydney, Australia

Kerekjarto, Margit von, Ph.D., Professor and Director Emeritus of Medical Psychology Department, University Clinic of Hamburg University, Eppendorf, Hamburg, Germany

Klussmann, Rudolf, M.D., Chief, Psychosomatics Department, University of Munich, Pittenkofer Strasse 8A, 8000 Munich, Germany

Köhle, Karl, M.D., Director and Professor of Psychosomatic Medicine, University of Cologne, Cologne, Germany

Küchler, Thomas, Ph.D., Medical Psychologist, Department of Medical Psychology, University Clinic of Hamburg University, Eppendorf, Hamburg, Germany

Linnemann, Ebbe, M.D., Emeritus Professor of Psychiatry, Copenhagen University, 267a Straadvejen, 2920 Charlottenlund, Denmark

Mitchell, Jeffrey T., Ph.D., Assistant Professor, Emergency Health Services Program, University of Maryland, Baltimore, Maryland, United States

Penny, Ronald, M.D., Professor of Clinical Immunology, University of New South Wales; Director, Centre for Immunology, St. Vincents Hospital, Sydney, Australia

Speidel, Hubert, M.D., Professor and Head of Psychotherapy and Psychosomatic Medicine, Christian-Albrechts Hospital, Kiel, Germany

Thyholdt, Reidar, Ph.D., Researcher, Research Centre for Occupational Health and Safety, University of Bergen, Bergen, Norway

Uexküll, Thure von, M.D., Professor Emeritus, University of Ulm. Residence: Sonnhalde 15, 7800 Freiburg, Germany

List of Claus Bahne Bahnson's Articles

1. Bahnson, C.B. Rhythmical Auditory Projection as a New Tool for Personality Assessment. Boston University School of Medicine. Psychosomatic Research Unit. August 1957.
1a. Abstract of above. *American Psychologist, 12*, 309, 1957.
2. Knapp, P.H. Bahnson, C.B. and Nemetz, S.J. Emotional Fluctuations in an Asthmatic Girl: A Pilot Study in Methods, Using Psychiatric and Psychological Observations, and a Model of Depressive Emotion. Boston University Medical School, 1958.
3. Bahnson, C.B. Conscious and Non-conscious Emotions and Their Relation to Ego Defenses, Regression and Symptom Formation: A New Technique of Assessment. Presented at Amer. Psychological Assoc., New York. August 1985.
4. Bahnson, C.B. A Tentative Psychodynamic Interpretation of Coronary Heart Disease. In Prog. Rep., Grant No. H-4257, NIH. Middlesex County Heart Study, Socio-Psychological Phase, 1960.
5. Bahnson, C.B. Psychological Obstacles to International Understanding. Summary of invited paper delivered at the United Nations on Nov. 17, 1961.
6. Bahnson, C.B. and Bahnson, M.B. Emotion vs. cognition as a core for personality theory. *Acta Psychol., 19*, 746-747, 1961.
7. Bahnson, C.B. and Wardwell, W.I. et al. Hartford Study: Social and psychological factors in heart disease. *Rev.*

and *Newsletter, Transcultural Research in Mental Health Problems,* No. 10, 60-61.
8. Bahnson, C.B. and Wardwell, W.I. The Coronary Personality, Results from the Middlesex Coronary Heart Study. 1961.
9. Knapp, P.H., and Bahnson, C.B. A longitudinal study of fantasy and mood in asthmatic patients. *Summaries of the Scientific Papers of the 117th Annual Meeting of the Amer. Psychiatric Assoc.,* 36-37, 1961.
10. Bahnson, C.B. and Wardwell, W.I. Parent constellation and psycho-sexual identification in male patients with myocardial infarction. *Psychological Reports, 10*(3), 831-852, 1962.
11. Wardwell, W.I., Bahnson, C.B., and Caron, H.S. Social and Psychological factors in coronary heart disease. *Journal of Health and Human Behavior,* 4, 154-165, 1963.
12. Bahnson, C.B. Therapeutic Teaching: A Climate for Creativity. Presented in symposium at the Amer. Personnel and Guidance Assoc. Conv. in Boston, Mass. Symposium Title: The Teacher as a Discordant Being: A Modern Dialectic. April 9, 1963.
13. Knapp, P.H. and Bahnson, C.B. The emotional field – A sequential study of mood and fantasy in two asthmatic patients. *Journal of Psychosomatic Medicine,* 25, 460-483, 1963.
14. Wardwell, W.I. and Bahnson, C.B. Problems encountered in behavioral science research in epidemiological studies. *American Journal of Public Health,* 54(6), 972-981, 1964.
15. Wardwell, W.I., Hyman, M. and Bahnson, C.B. Stress and coronary heart disease in three field studies. *Journal of Chronic Diseases,* 17, 73-84, 1964.
16. Bahnson, C.B. and Bahnson, M.B. Denial and repression of primitive impulses and of disturbing emotions in patients with malignant neoplasms. In D.M. Kissen and L.L. LeShan (Eds.), *Psychosomatic Aspects of Neoplastic Disease.* Lippincott, Phila., 42-62, 1964.

17. Bahnson, C.B. and Bahnson, M.B. Cancer as an alternative to psychosis: A theoretical model of somatic and psychologic regression. In D.M. Kissen and L.L. LeShan (Eds.), *Psychosomatic Aspects of Neoplastic Disease.* Lippincott, Phila., PA, 184-202, 1964.
18. Bahnson, C.B. Emotional reactions to internally and externally derived threat of annihilation. In G.H. Grosser, H. Wechsler, and M. Greenblatt (Eds.), *The Threat of Impending Disaster.* MIT Press, 251-280, 1964.
18a. Bahnson, C.B., and Wardwell, W.I. Coronary personality Patterns. Paper presented at the Eastern Psychological Assoc. Annual Meeting, Atlantic City, New Jersey, April, 1965.
19. Bahnson, C.B. Panel discussion: Retrospects and Prospects. In C.B. Bahnson and D.M. Kissen (Eds.), Psychophysiological Aspects of Cancer. *Annals NYAS, 125*(3), 1028-1055, 1966.
20. Bahnson, C.B. and Bahnson, M.B. Role of the ego defenses: denial and repression in the etiology of malignant neoplasm. In C.B. Bahnson and D.M. Kissen (Eds.), Psychophysiological Aspects of Cancer. *Annals NYAS, 125*(3), 827-845, 1966.
21. Bahnson, C.B. and Wardwell, W.I. Personality factors predisposing to myocardial infarction. In *Psychosomatic Medicine, Proc. of the first Internat. Conf. of the Academy of Psychosom. Med.*, Excerpta Med., Int'l. Congress Series No. 134, 249-256, 1966.
22. Bahnson, C.B. Gegenwartige Strömungen in der Psychosomatischen Forschung und Skizzierung eines Komplementaren Theoretischen Modells. In: *Therapie über das Nervensystem.* Hippokrates Verlag, Wiesbaden, 6, 11-44, 1966.
23. Bahnson, C.B. New mysticism, old bottles. Review of Herbert Read's "The Forms of Things Unknown." *Contemporary Psychology, 11*(7), 333-335, 1966.
24. Bahnson, C.B. Identity, Creativity and Conformity. In *Eastern Pennsylvania Psychiatric Institute Forum* and *Institute of Pennsylvania Hospital Press.* Philadelphia, Pennsylvania. 1966.

25. Bahnson, C.B., Ifarraguerri, A., and Cornelison, F.S. Personality and self-image in hemophilic patients. In *Proc. of the IV World Congress of Psychiatry*, Excerpta Medica. Int'l. Congress Series No. 150, 2752-2754, 1966.
26. Bahnson, C.B. Psychiatrisch-Psychologische Aspekte bei Krebspatienten. In *Proc. of 73rd Convention of the German Soc. for Int'l. Med.* Bergman Publ., Munich, 536-550, 1967.
27. Bahnson, C.B. Der Tumorkranke in der ärztlichen Praxis. *Proc. of 73rd Convention of the German Soc. for Int'l. Med.*, Bergman Publ., Munich, 555-557, 1967.
28. Bahnson, C.B. Psychodynamische Prozesse und Personlichkeitsfaktoren bei Krebskranken. *Prophylaxe. Int'l. J. of Prophylactic Med. and Soc. Hygiene*, 6(2), 17-26, 1967.
29. Wardwell, W.I., Hyman, M. and Bahnson, C.B. Socio-environmental antecedents to coronary heart disease in 87 white males. *Social Science and Medicine*, 2, 165-183, 1968.
30. Bahnson, C.B. and Bahnson, M.B. Repressed ego, flat emotions – cancer link. *Psychiatric Progress*, 3(4), 8, 1968.
31. Bahnson, C.B. Body and self-images associated with audio-visual self-confrontation. *Journal of Nervous and Mental Disease*, 148(3), 262-280, 1969.
32. Bahnson, M.B. and Bahnson, C.B. Ego defenses in cancer patients. In C.B. Bahnson, (Ed.), Second Conf. on Psychophysiological Aspects of Cancer. *Annals NYAS*, 164(2), 546-559, 1969.
33. Bahnson, C.B. Psychophysiological complementarity in malignancies: past work and future vistas. In C.B. Bahnson, (Ed.), Second Conf. on Psychophysiological Aspects of Cancer. *Annals NYAS*, 164(2), 590-610, 1969.
34. Bahnson, C.B. David M. Kissens work: In memoriam. In C.B. Bahnson (Ed.) Second Conf. on Psychophysiological Aspects of Cancer. *Annals NYAS*, 164(2), 313-318, 1969.
35. Bahnson, C.B. Theoretical Psychophysiological Considerations, General Discussion. In C.B. Bahnson (Ed.) ,

Second Conf. on Psychophysiological Aspects of Cancer. *Annals NYAS*, 163(2), 590-610, 1969.
36. Comment. Ibid, 430-1969.
37. Bahnson, C.B. Integration and evaluation of current psychophysiological approaches to cancer. Panel discussion 3: The psychological approach. In C.B. Bahnson, (Ed.), Second Conf. on Psychophysiological Aspects of Cancer. *Annals NYAS*, 164(2), 628-34, 1969.
38. Bahnson, C.B. Der Psycho-physiologische Ansatz zu Krebs. *Der Mensch und Die Technik*, March 5, 1970.
39. Bahnson, C.B. Basic epistemological considerations regarding psychosomatic processes and their application to current psychophysiological cancer research. *International Journal of Psychobiol.*, 1, 57-69, 1970.
40. Bahnson, C.B. Theory and research on the complementarity of regression in somatic and behavioral disorganization. APA, Miami, Fla., Sept. 1970.
41. Bahnson, C.B., Wardwell, W.I., Bahnson, M.B., and Luck, P.W. Psychological characteristics of male patients with primary myocardial infarction. Academy of Psychosomatic Medicine. Hamilton, Bermuda, 1970.
42. Bahnson, C.B., Bahnson, M.B., and Wardwell, W.I. A psychologic study of cancer patients. American Psychosomatic Society, Denver, Colo., April 1971.
43. Bahnson, C.B. The psychological aspects of cancer. The American Cancer Society's Thirteenth Science Writers' Seminar. Phoenix, AZ., April 1971.
44. Bahnson, C.B. To like and to be like: Object relationship and identification in schizophrenia. Proc. of the Fourth Inter. Symposium on Psychotherapy of Schizophrenia, Turku, Finland, 1971. Excerpta Medica, pp. 38-45, 1971.
45. Bahnson, C.B. The theory of psychophysiological complementarity: Applied to cancer and coronary heart disease. *Proc. of the XVII Congress of Applied Psychology*. Liege, Belgium, July 1971. Editest, Brussels, Belgium, 1971.
46. Wardwell, W.I. and Bahnson, C.B. Pattern A, stress and

anxiety in an epidemiologic study of myocardial infarction. Fourth Annual Meeting of the Society for Epidemiologic Research, Atlanta, Ga., May 1971.
47. Bahnson, C.B., Bahnson, M.B., and Wardwell, W.I. A psychologic study of cancer patients. (Abstract), *Psychosomatic Medicine*, 33(5), 466-467, 1971.
48. Bahnson, C.B. Psychoanalytic theory and problems of contemporary youth. Proc. of the New York Academy of Psychoanalysis, New York, Dec. 1971. *Science and Psychoanalysis*, Vol XXI, 237-242, 1972.
49. Bahnson, C.B. Psychoanalytic and family therapy studies of drug abusers and their families. Presented at the joint session of the Academy of Psychoanalysis and the American Ortho. Assoc., Detroit, Mich., April 1972.
50. Wardwell, W.I., and Bahnson, C.B. A study of stress and coronary heart disease in an urban population. *Bulletin of the N.Y. Academy of Medicine, Second Series*, 49, 521-531, 1973.
51. Bahnson, C.B. Identification, differentiation and complementarity in schizophrenic families. Presented at symposium on Schizophrenia and the Family: Research and Theory. Phila., Pa., April 1973.
52. Wardwell, W.I. and Bahnson, C.B. Behavioral variables and myocardial infarction in the Southeastern Connecticut Heart Study. *Journal of Chronic Disease*, 26, 447-461, 1973.
53. Bahnson, C.B. Projective technitherapy. Review of Joseph E. Shorr's "Psycho-Imagination Therapy." *Contemporary Psychology*, 19, 326-328, 1974.
54. Miller, B., Sheehan, M., and Bahnson, C.B. Psychosocial aspects of drug abuse. In W. White Jr. and R.F. Albano (Eds.), *North American Symposium on Drugs and Drug Abuse*. North American Publishing Co., Phila., Pa., 96-104, 1974.
55. Bahnson, C.B. Adolescent turmoil: Interactions in the family system. In D.W. Abse, E.M. Nash, L.M.R. Louden (Eds.). *Marital and Sexual Counseling in Medical Practice*. Harper and Row, Hagerstown, Md., 310-334, 1974.

56. Bahnson, C.B., Bahnson, M.B., Siskin, B., Luck, P.W., and Wardwell, W.I. The interaction of smoking and personality characteristics in healthy subjects and seriously ill patients. Annual Meeting of the Eastern Psychological Assoc., Phila., Pa., April 1974.
57. Bartuska, D.G., Smith J., and Bahnson, C.B. Psychological correlates of thyrotoxicosis. (Abstract) *Clinical Research*, XXII, (3), 335A, April 1974.
58. Bahnson, C.B. Adolescents and their parents, a dynamic systems theoretical approach. 8th Int'l. Congress of the Int'l. Assoc. for Child Psychiatry and Allied Professions. Phila., Pa., July 1974.
59. Bahnson, C.B. and Bahnson, M.B. Personality variables and life experiences predicting specific disease syndromes. American Psychological Assoc. New Orleans, La., Sept. 1974.
60. Behavioral factors associated with the etiology of physical disease. *American Journal of Public Health*, 64(11), 1033-1055, 1974. Six papers presented at the APHA symposium on behavioral factors and the etiology of physical disease; organized, chaired, and edited by C.B. Bahnson, Houston, TX, October, 1970: Bahnson, C.B. Introduction; and, Epistemiological perspectives of physical disease from the psychodynamic point of view.
61. Bahnson, C.B. Epistemological perspectives of physical disease from the psychodynamic point of view. *American Journal of Public Health*, 64(11), 1034-1040, 1974.
62. Bahnson, C.B. Life stress, personality, disease, and death. *Eastern Penn. Psychiatric Inst. Science News Quarterly*, 1(1), 2-3, Summer, 1974.
63. Bahnson, C.B. Life threatening illness: Mental health treatment and training programs. *Eastern Penn. Psychiatric Inst. Science News Quarterly*, 1(3), 1 & 9, Winter 1975.
64. Bahnson, C.B. and Smith, K. Autonomic changes in a multiple personality. (Abstract). *Psychosomatic Medicine*, 37(1), 85-86, 1975.
65. Bahnson, C.B. Psychologic and emotional issues in can-

cer: the psychotherapeutic care of the cancer patient. In *Seminars in Oncology*. Grune and Stratton, New York 2(4), 293-309, 1975.
66. Bahnson, C.B. Emotional and personality characteristics of cancer patients. In A.I. Sutnick and P.F. Engstrom (Eds.), *Oncologic Medicine: Clinical Topics and Practical Management*. Univ. Park Press, Balt., MD, 357-378, 1976.
67. APA Task Force on Health Research. (C.B. Bahnson, co-contributor). Contributions of psychology to health research: patterns, problems, and potentials. *American Psychologist*, 31(4), 263-274, 1976.
68. Bahnson, C.B. A Psychosomatic Approach to Selected Epidemiologic Studies of Cancer. Eastern Penn. Psychiatric Inst., Nov. 1976.
69. Bahnson, C.B. Thoughts on psychosomatic issues. *The Academy*. (The Amer. Acad. of Psychoanalysis), 21(2), 6-8, May 1977.
70. Cramer, I., Blohmke, M., Bahnson, C.B., Bahnson, M.B., Scherg, H., Weinhold, M. Psychosoziale Faktoren und Krebs: Untersuchung von 80 Frauen mit einem psychosozialen Fragenbogen. *Munch. med. Wschr.*, 119(43), 1387-1392, 1977.
71. Baskin, S.I., Klekotka, S.J., Smith, J., Bahnson, C.B., Bartuska, D.G. Behavioral characteristics and platelet taurine levels in patients with thyroid disease (Abstract). The Endocrine Society, June 8-10, 1977.
72. Bahnson, C.B. The psychoanalytic view of the family system with regard to the psychopathology of the adolescent. Joint session of the American Ortho. Assoc. and the Acad. of Psychoanalysis, New York City, April 1977.
73. Bahnson, C.B. Presidente de seance: Problems psychologiques poses par la prevention des cancers O.R.L. In R. Fresco and J. Extremet (Eds.), *Psychologie et Cancer*. Discussions et Tables Rondes. Institut J. Paoli-l. Calmettes, 5-9. 1977.
74. Bahnson, C.B. Multiple Personality and Altered Ego States; Clinical and Theoretical Implications in Terms of

Psychodynamics, Family Experience, and Anxiety about Non-Existence and Death. Delivered at the VI Int'l. Forum of Psychoanalysis, Berlin, West Germany, Aug. 17-21, 1977.

75. Bahnson, C.B. Stress Psychologique familial et probleme des antecedents psychoaffectifs du cancer. In R. Fresco and J. Extremet (Eds.), *Psychologie et Cancer.* Masson, Paris, 13-16, 1978.

76. Bahnson, C.B. Psychotherapie chez les malades cancereux en phase terminale. In R. Fresco and J. Extremet (Eds.), *Psychologie et Cancer.* Masson, Paris, 97-99, 1978.

77. Bahnson, C.B. Characteristics of a psychotherapeutic treatment program for cancer. In H.E. Nieburgs (Ed.), *Prevention and Detection of Cancer,* Part 1, Vol. 2, Marcel Dekker, New York, 2309-2312, 1978.

78. Bahnson, C.B. Problemi psicologici ed emotivi in oncologia: il trattamento psicoterapeutico del malato neoplastico. *Aggiornamenti in Oncologia clinica* (Rome), 4(1), 19-52, 1978.

79. Bahnson, C.B. Psychological and Social Dimensions of Dealing with the Very Sick Cancer Patient. Address delivered at the Seminar at the Woodrow Wilson Center at the Smithsonian Institution, Wash., D.C., June 28, 1978.

80. Bahnson, C.B. Dying, death and the family. *Interaction,* 2(3), 155-164, Fall 1979.

81. Bahnson, M.B. and Bahnson, C.B. Development of a psychosocial screening questionnaire for cancer. *Cancer Detection and Prevention,* 2(2), Marcel Dekker, New York, 295-305, 1979.

82. Bahnson, C.B. An Historical Family Systems Approach to Coronary Heart Disease and Cancer. In K.E. Schaefer, U. Stave, W. Blankenburg (Eds.), *A New Image of Man in Medicine.* Vol. III Individuation Process in Biographical Aspects of Disease. Futura Publishing Co., Inc., Mount Kisco, N.Y., 145-191, 1979.

83. Bahnson, C.B. Das Krebsproblem in Psychomatischer

Dimension. In Thure von Uexküll (Ed.), *Lechrbuch der Psychosomatischen Medizin.* Urban and Schwarzenberg, Munich, 685-698, 1979.
84. Bahnson, C.B. Stress and Cancer: The State of the Art. Second Annual Conf. and Workshops on Psychosomatic Disorders: Medicine Looks at Stress. The Dept. of Psychiatry and Human Behavior, Jefferson Medical College of Thomas Jefferson Univ., April 27, 1979.
85. Bahnson, C.B. The Psychologic Approach to Breast Cancer. Paper delivered at the Second Breast Cancer Working Conf. held by the European Organization for Research on Treatment of Cancer, Breast Cancer Cooperative Group, Copenhagen, Denmark, June 2, 1979.
86. Bahnson, C.B. Family of the Terminal Patient: Psychological and Emotional Issues. In *Psykoterapeutisk Workshop.* Copenhagen Univ. Denmark, Vol. 23, August 1979.
87. Bahnson, C.B. Psychosocial Factors and Cancer. Scientific Conv. of the German Society for Social Medicine, Heidelberg, West Germany, Sept. 27, 1979.
88. Bahnson, C.B. The Psychological Approach to the Cancer Patient. Health for a New Age Seminar: New Approaches to Cancer. The Royal Society of Medicine, London, Nov. 1979.
89. Bahnson, C.B. Intrapsychic Reactions to Aging. Weiss-English Psychosomatic Symposium, Phila., Pa., Nov. 17, 1979. Also on audio cassette tape and abstracted in *Audio-Digest, 9*(2), Jan. 28, 1980.
90. Bahnson, C.B. Nonverbal Behavior in Psychotherapy. In S.A. Corson and E.O. Corson (Eds.), *Ethology and Nonverbal Communication in Mental Health.* Pergamon Press, Oxford, England, 123-134, 1980.
91. Bahnson, C.B. The Use of Imagery and Altered States in Patients with Terminal Disease. American Psychiatric Assoc., Symposium: Altered States in Serious Illness and Dying, San Francisco, CA, May 3-9, 1980.
92. Bahnson, C.B. Psychotherapy as a Psychologic Discipline. In M. Dongier and E.D. Wittkower (Eds.), *Divergent*

Views in Psychiatry. Harper and Row, New York, 69-95, 1981.
93. Bahnson, C.B. Psychosomatic Issues in Cancer. In R.L. Gallon (Ed). The Psychosomatic Approach to Illness. Elsevier-North Holland, New York, 53-87, 1982.
94. Bahnson, C.B. Stress and Cancer: The State of the Art. In Psychosomatics, Part 1, 21(12), 975-981, Dec. 1980; Part II, 22(3), 207-220, March 1981.
95. Bahnson, C.B. Disability in Classical Myth and Modern Society. Presented at workshop/seminar: The Woodrow Wilson Int'l. Center for Scholars, Smithsonian Institute, Wash., D.C. May 13, 1981.
96. Bahnson, C.B. Key Psychologic Markers in the Etiology and Psychotherapy of Cancer Patients. 6th World Congress of the Int'l. College of Psychosomatic Medicine, Montreal, Quebec, Canada, Sept. 15, 1981.
97. Bahnson, C.B. Family development, Somatic Illness, and Needs in Psychologic Treatment. 6th World Congress of the Int'l. College of Psychosomatic Medicine, Montreal, Quebec, Canada, Sept. 17, 1981.
98. Bahnson, C.B. Systems Concepts in Group and Family Therapy. In M. Pines and L. Rafaelsen (Eds.), The Individual and the Group, Vol. 1, Plenum Publishing Corp., 157-168, 1982.
99. Bahnson, C.B. The Psychosomatic Approach to Gynecologic Cancers. In H.J. Prill and M. Stauber (Eds.), Advances in Psychosomatic Obstetrics and Gynecology, Springer-Verlag, Berlin, Heidelberg, New York, 175-285, 1982.
100. Bahnson, C.B. Treating Family Illness Systems: Heart Disease and Cancer. UCLA Extension Conf.: Beyond the Relaxation Response: Self-Regulation Mechanisms and Clinical Strategies, UCLA School of Medicine, Los Angeles, Ca., Feb. 26-27, 1983.
101. Bahnson, C.B. Individual and Family Response to External and Internal Stress. Seventh World Congress of Psychiatry. Vienna, July 11-16, 1983.
102. Bahnson, C.B. The State of the Arts in Psycho-oncology.

Seventh World Congress of the Int'l. College of Psychosomatic Medicine, Hamburg, July 22-27, 1983.
103. Bahnson, C.B. Psychological Aspects of Cancer. In Y.H. Pilch, T.K. Das Grupta (Eds.), *Surgical Oncology.* McGraw-Hill Book Co., New York, 231-253, 1984.
104. Bahnson, C.B. The Psychosomatic Approach in Medical Practice. Keynote address to the Int'l. Balint Society, Ascona, Switzerland, April 1, 1984.
105. Bahnson, C.B. Research on Family Therapy and Hypertension. Presented at the Annual Meeting of the American Family Therapy Assoc., New York City, June 14-17, 1984.
106. Bahnson, C.B. and Engelman, S. Questions Concerning the Psychologic Impact and Traetment of AIDS. Paper presented at the Annual Convention of the American Psychological Assoc. in Toronto, Canada, Aug. 24-28, 1984.
107. Bahnson, C.B. Integration and Disintegration of Personality: Multiple Personality and Altered Egostates. Presented at the Annual Convention of the American Psychological Assoc. in Toronto, Canada, Aug. 24-28, 1984.
108. Bahnson, C.B. The Case of AIDS: Immunologic Linkage Between Psychologic State and Cellular Pathology. Presented at the Annual Meeting of the Academy of Psychosomatic Medicine in Phila., PA, Nov. 11-14, 1984.
109. Bahnson, C.B. Family Therapy in Serious and Terminal Illness. Presented in seminar at the AFTA Annual Meeting in New York City, June 14-17, 1984. In *Psychiatry*, Vol. 5, 449-455. P.Pichot, P. Berner, R. Wolf and K. Thau, (Eds.), Plenum Publishing Corp., 1985.
110. Bahnson, C.B. The Phenomenology of Responses to External and Internal Threats of Annihilation in War and Disease. The Third Int'l. Conf. on Psychological Stress and Adjustment in Time of War and Peace, Tel Aviv, Isreal, Jan. 3, 1983. In *Psychiatry*, Vol. 4, 389-395. P.Pichot, P. Berner, R. Wolf and K. Thau, (Eds.), Plenum Publishing Corp., 1985.
111. Bremond, A., Kune, G., and Bahnson, C.B. Psychoso-

matic Factors in Breast Cancer Patients, Results of a Case Control Study. In *Journal of Psychosomatic Obstetrics and Gynecology*, 5:127-136, 1986.

112. Bahnson, C.B. Separation and Loss in Women with Mastectomies. Presented at the Annual Meeting of the American Academy of Psychoanalysis, Dallas, Texas, May 16-19, 1985.
113. Bahnson, C.B. Somatic Illness in the Family: The Scorpion Stings Itself. Presented at the VII Int"l. Delphic Symposium on Family Therapy, Athens, Greece, April 22-25, 1985.
114. Bahnson, C.B. Life Threatening Disease: Individuation and the Family. In *AFTA Proceedings: Abstracts of the Seventh Annual Meeting of the American Family Therapy Assoc.*, San Diego, CA, June 12-16, 1985.
115. Bahnson, C.B. The Clinical Relationship Between Interpersonal Experience, Depressive Emotions and Immunologic Response to Disease. Presented at the VIIIth Annual Conf. on Psychosomatic Disorders, Oct. 24-25, 1985, Jefferson Medical College, Phila., PA.
116. Bahnson, C.B. Das Krebsproblem in Psychosomatischer Dimension. In *Psychosomatische Medizin*, 889-909 (erweiterte Auflage), Verlag Urban und Schwarzenberg, München, Wien, Baltimore, 1986.
117. Bahnson, C.B. The Impact of Life Threatening Illness on the Family – The Impact of the Family on Illness – An Overview. In *Family and Life Threatening Illness*, Family Nursing Series, Vol. 1, 21-44, L. Wright and M. Leahey, (Eds.), Springhouse Publishers, PA, 1987.
118. Bahnson, C.B. Trennungs- und Verlusterlebnisse bei Frauen mit Mastektomie. In *Psychother. med. Psychol. 36*, 25-31, Georg Thieme Verlag Stuttgart, New York, 1986.
119. Bahnson, C.B. Körperliche Krankheit in der Familie: Der Skorpion Sticht Sich Selbst. In *Perspektiven*, Journal für Wissenschaft, Kultur und Praxis in der Medizin, Universität Witten/Herdecke, Vol. 2, 36-39, Jan. 1986.
120. Bahnson, C.B., Hudson, D., Mallios, R., Blohmke, M. and

Scherg, H. Psychosocial Predictors of Breast Cancer. Presented at the 1986 Annual Convention of the American Psychosomatic Society, Baltimore.
121. Bahnson, C.B. Politische Folgen von individuellen psychodynamischen Konflikten. Präsentiert auf dem Symposium "Individuelle und gesellschaftliche Aspekte der Tiefenpsychologie", Christian-Albrechts-Universität, Kiel, 06. Dezember 1986.
122. Bahnson, C.B. Körperliche Krankheit in der Familie: Der Skorpion Sticht Sich Selbst. In *Psychosomatische Störungen*, 67-79, J. Derbolowsky. und I. Middendorf (Eds.), E. Fischer Verlag, Heidelberg, 1986.
123. Bahnson, C.B. Familie, Objektverlust, Abwehrstil und Spätfolgen bei Krankheit und Sozialpathologie. In *Beiträge zur Psychoonkologie*, 5-40, Österreichische Gesellschaft für Psychoonkologie (Eds.), Facultas Universitätsverlag, Wien, 1988.
124. Bahnson, C.B. The Forgotten Language of Artistic Symbol and Biological Symptom Formation. In *Incontro Con Erich Fromm*, 71-78; Pier Lorenzo Eletti (Ed.), Edizioni Medicea, Florence, 1988.
125. Bahnson, C.B. Biographie und Tumorerkrankung I. Herdecker Herbstkongreß, 25.-26. September 1987. In *Onkologie im Spannungsfeld konventioneller und ganzheitlicher Betrachtung, Aktuelle Onkologie*, Vol. 48, 78-93, P.F. Matthiessen, C.H.-Tautz (Eds.), Zuckschwerdt Verlag München, Bern, Wien , San Francisco, 1988.
126. Bahnson, C.B. Familie, Abwehrstil und Spätfolgen bei Krankheit und Sozialpathologie, 16. Norddeutsche Psychotherapie-Tage, Lübeck, 3.-9. Oktober 1987.
127. Bahnson, C.B. Therapeutische Aspekte im Umgang mit Sterbenden und deren Familie, "Der Schwierige Fall", Aggression und Trauer in der therapeutischen und pädischen Arbeit, 6. wissenschaftliche Arbeitstagung veranstaltet von der Deutschen Gesellschaft für Psychotherapie und Psychopädie e.V. (PSG), Berlin, 9.-11. Oktober 1987.

128. Bahnson, C.B. Zeitgenössische Psychosomatische Ansätze zu Krebskrankheiten und anderen schweren chronischen Krankheiten. Jahrestagung der Österreichischen Gesellschaft für Psychoonkologie, Bad Ischl, 13.-15. November 1987.
129. Bahnson, C.B. Familie, Objektverlust, Abwehrstil und Spätfolgen. In *Beiträge zur Psychoonkologie*, 5-40, Hrsg. ÖGPO Facultas Verlag, Wien, 1988.
130. Bahnson, C.B. Psychosomatik chronischer köperlicher Erkrankungen. In *Zukunftsaufgaben der Psychosomatischen Medizin*, 73-83, Speidel, H. und Strauss, B. (Eds.), Springer-Verlag, Berlin, Heidelberg, New York, 1989.
131. Bahnson, C.B. Psychodynamischer Zugang zum AIDs-Kranken, psychosomatische und psychotherapeutische Aspekte. In *Zur Klinik und Praxis der Aids-Krankheit*, 25-31, R. Klußmann, F.-D. Goebel (Eds.), Springer-Verlag, Berlin, Heidelberg, New York, 1989.
132. Bahnson, C.B. Kunst und Therapie. Festvortrag (keynote) zum 5. Jahreskongreß der IAACT, Salzburg, 6.10.1989.
133. Bahnson, C.B. Familientherapie bei Krebskranken – Unter Berücksichtigung von Objektverlust und Verdrängung. In *Der Krebskranke*, 70-82. R. Klußmann u. B. Emmerich (Eds.), Springer-Verlag, Berlin, Heidelberg, New York, 1990.
134. Bahnson, C.B. Therapie von Lebenskrisen zur Bewältigung chronischer Krankheiten. In *Praktische Psychotherapie*, J. Derbolowsky und U. Derbolowsky (Eds.), V.f.M. Fischer, Heidelberg, 1990.
135. Bahnson, C.B. Bestzung und Verlust von Person und Objekt. In ÖGPO (Ed.), *Beiträge zur Psychoonkologie*, Band 5, Facultas Verlag, Wien, 1990.
136. Kune, G.A., Kune, S., Watson, L.F., Bahnson C.B. Personality as a risk factor in large Bowel cancer: data from the Melbourne Colorectal Cancer Study *Psychological Medicine*, Vol. 21, 29-41, 1991.

137. Bahnson, C.B. Die Bedeutung der Psychoonkologie in der Nachsorge Festvortrag anläßlich der 12. Gesamtösterreichischen Arbeitstagung der Frauenselbsthilfe nach Krebs in Österreich vom 10. bis 13.10.1991, Wolfsberg, Kärnten.
138. Bahnson, C.B., Gallmeier, W.N., Kappauf, H.W., von Kleist, S., Munk, K. (Eds.), Psychoneuroimmunologie und Krebs (PNI and cancer). Monograph from Onkologie, Supplement No. 1, Vol. 14, Karger, Basel, August 1991.
139. Bahnson, C.B. Psychosomatisch-systemische Ansätze im Allgemeinen Krankenhaus In.: Jahrbuch der Psychoonkologie, Österreichische Gesellschaft für Psychoonkologie (Eds.), Springer-Verlag, Wien, New York, 1992 (in press)
140. Bahnson, C.B. Medical, Therapeutic and Political Systems in Transition: The New Era. Opening Paper at the First Baltic Sea Conference on Psychosomatics and Psychotherapy, Kiel 1992 (in press)
141. Bahnson, C.B. Cancer as a Psychosomatic Disease. Paper delivered at the First Baltic Sea Conference, Kiel 1992.
142. Bahnson, C.B. Families as producers and sufferers from somatic disease. Paper delivered at the first Baltic Sea Conference, Kiel 1992.
143. Bahnson, C.B. Quality of life with Cancer, Paper delivered at German Red Cross Convention, Nov. 28.1992, Kiel. (in press)
144. Bahnson, C.B. Die psycho-analytische Symbolik des Körpers. Vortrag auf der Tagung "Der Körper als Problem des älteren Menschen" – Rehabilitation und Geriatrie – der Sozial- und Arbeitsmedizinischen Akademie Baden-Württemberg e.V. in Verbindung mit der Universität Ulm. Medizinische Gesellschaft Glotterbad e.V. 18.06.-19.06.92

Index (by author)

A

Ackerman, N. W., 119, 120, 135
Adams, J. E., 10, 26
Adams, L. E., 180
Adena, Michael, 178
Ader, Robert, xx
Adler, Alfred, 101, 102
Adler, G., 81, 83
Alexander, F., xiv, 119, 135
Allison, E. J., 32, 44
Andrews, F. M., 57, 65
Andrews, G., 158, 165, 183
Aslop, Stewart, 142, 143, 144, 149, 151, 152, 155

B

Bahnson, Claus Bahne, xi, xii, xiv, xvi, xix, xx, xxii, xxvi, 3, 26, 53, 54, 65, 70, 71, 83, 90, 93, 105, 106, 108, 109, 116, 133, 135, 159, 179, 203, 204, 219, 220, 222, 227-242
Bahnson, Linda Weiss, xxvi
Bahnson, M. B., 65, 222, 227, 228, 229, 230, 231, 233, 234, 235
Baker, R. J., 179
Balint, M., 214, 223
Barker, D., 6, 29
Barr, Epstein, 159
Bartrop, Roger W., 158, 161, 163, 165, 166, 167, 169, 179, 180, 182, 225

Bartrop-Schneider, Sue, 178
Bartuska, D. G., 232
Baskin, S. I., 234
Bateson, G., 135, 213, 223
Bauer, G., 74, 83
Baumann, Thomas, 68
Bayliss, 206
Becker, H., 89, 93
Becker, R., 4, 5, 26
Beckett, A., 81, 83
Beckmann, D., 10, 26
Beecher, xiv
Begemann-Deppe, M., 187, 199
Behrens, M. L., 120, 135
Benedetti, Gaetano, 46, 47, 48, 50, 53, 54
Benjamin, B., 161, 183
Bent, D. H., 35, 44
Berah, E. F., 32, 44
Bergmann, A., 223
Bernard, Claude, xiv, 206
Bertalanffy, L. von, 120, 125, 135, 223
Bidder, Friedrich, xiii
Biggs, J. C., 180
Bilek, Hans Peter, 94, 225
Binger, Carl A., 119, 135
Bjorneboe, Jens, xxii
Blades, B. C., 59, 66
Bliesener, T., 189, 190, 200
Blohmke, M., 160, 182, 234
Bloomfield, H., 104, 117
Böck, D., 190, 201
Boll, Annegret, 3, 5, 6, 7, 10, 26, 28, 30, 225
Booth, Gotthard, 51, 54, 55

Borysenko, Joan, xx
Bowman, F. O., 8, 27
Bradbury, L., 32, 45
Bremond, A., 239
Breslow, N. E., 175, 180
Brodsky, B., 140, 155
Bromberg, W., 141, 155
Brown, J. S., 6, 7, 8, 22, 25, 26
Brown, M. B., 180
Brown, S. A., 181
Bruch, Hilde, 119, 126, 135
Buchholz, M. B., 74, 83
Bulloch, Karen, xx
Burt, R. S., 56, 66

C

Caldwell, C., 181
Camerino, M., 182
Campbell, A. P., 57, 58, 59, 66
Campbell, D. T., 63, 66
Cannon, Walter B., xiii, 119, 135
Caron, H. S., 228
Carroll, B. J., 181
Caruso, A. I., 100, 102
Clement, U., 69, 84
Charcot, Jean Martin, xviii
Cohen, R., 10, 26
Cohn, A. F., 119, 135
Comstock, G. W., 161, 181
Congalton, A. A., 164, 180
Converse, P. E., 57, 66
Cooper, D. A., 165, 180
Cooperband, S. R., 166, 180
Cornelison, A., 119, 136
Cornelison, F. S., 230
Cousins, Norman, xi, 107, 117, 225
Cox, P. R., 161, 180
Craig, A. R., 180
Cramer, I., 160, 182, 234
Craucher, Lisa, 178
Crawford, June, 178

D

Dahme, B., 4, 6, 7, 26, 27, 28, 30
Dahme, G., 6, 7, 22, 26
Dahme, P., 4, 29
Daniel House, J., 181
Davies-Osterkamp, S., 6, 27, 29
Davis, K. L., 182, 183
Dean, C., 160, 180
Dell Orto, A., 108, 117
Demi, A. S., 32, 44
Deneke, F. W., 186, 201
Descartes, Rene, 215
Deutsch, Felix, 119, 135
Dietz, A., 8, 28
Dillon, Kathleen, xx
Diwell, A. E., 6, 29
Dixon, W. J., 175, 180
Dostoevsky, Fedor, xxii
Dreikurs, R., 95, 102
Dunbar, H. Flanders, 119, 135
Durham, T. W., 32, 39, 44
Dyregrov, Atle, 31, 41, 42, 44, 225

E

Ehlich, K., 189, 196, 199, 200
Ehrenberg, 138
Ehrenfels, Ch. von, 207, 223
Eissler, K. R., 101, 102, 140, 141, 154, 156
Elkes, Joel, xx
Engel, George, xiv, xx
Engelman, L., 180
Engelman, Suzanne R., v, xxvi, 104, 105, 117, 225, 238
English, O. S., 191, 202
Ersland, S., 32, 45

F

Fahrenberg, J., 10, 27
Fanshel, D., 188, 201

Index (by author)

Fehlenberg, Dirk, 184, 225
Ferenci, S., 213, 223
Firman, J., 105, 109, 117
Flader, D., 196, 200
Fleck, Steven, 118, 119, 122, 132, 135, 136, 225
Flemming, B., 4, 27, 29, 30
Foad, B. S. I., 163, 180
Forcier, Lina, 158, 180, 225
Ford, J. R., 161, 180
Fornari, F., 214, 223
Frank, K. A., 8, 27
Frazer, A. G., 32, 33, 45
Freud, Anna, 148
Freud, Sigmund, xviii, xxii, 48, 52, 55, 74, 95, 119, 135, 138, 139,154, 156, 204, 205, 206, 208, 209, 210, 213, 221, 223
Friedson, E., 186, 200

G

Galen, Claudius, xi
Garner, W., 181
Gauguin, Paul, xxi
Gerson, E. M., 56, 66
Gillin, J. C., 181
Glaser, Ronald, xx, 159, 180, 181
Goethe, J. W., 101, 102
Good, R. A., 218, 223
Gorsuch, R. L., 164, 169, 171, 183
Götze, P., 4, 7, 10, 27, 28, 29, 30
Grant, I., 181
Grauhan, A., 190, 201
Greden, J., 181
Greene, W. A., 156
Greer, S., 160, 178, 180, 181, 182, 183
Groddeck, G., 48, 55
Grodzicki, W. D., 196, 200
Gück, J., 188, 189, 200
Gunther, John, 142, 143, 150, 156
Gunther, Johnny, 142-143, 149, 151

Gutzwiller, F., 74, 83

H

Hackett, T. P., 140, 141, 156
Haley, J., 135
Hamilton, M., 169, 171, 181
Hampel, R., 10, 27
Hancock, K., 180
Hansen, P., 166, 183
Harlow, H. F., 219, 223
Harmann, H., 213, 223
Heidegger, Martin, 138
Heller, S. S., 5, 7, 8, 22, 24, 27
Helsing, K. J., 161, 181
Henry, J. P., 223
Herberman, R. B., 181
Hertz, Dan G., 137, 226
Hesse, Hermann, 101, 102
Heusser, R., 74, 78, 83
Heyer, xiv
Hinkle, L. E., 119, 135
Hoffman, F., 183
Holliday, J. R., 181
Hollos, I., 97, 102
Hull, C. H., 35, 45
Huse-Kleinstoll, G., 4, 6, 7, 22, 24, 26, 27, 28, 29, 30
Huygen, F. J., 119, 136
Hyman, M., 228, 230

I

Ifarraguerri, A., 230
Ilinitch, R. C., 32, 44
Irwin, M., 177, 181

J

Jackson, D., 135, 165, 181
Jacob, Wolfgang, 46, 47, 52, 55, 226
Jährig, C., 186, 200
Jenkins, C. D., 6, 30

Jenkins, J. G., 35, 45
Jennerich, R. T., 180
Jenson, J., 177, 181
Johnson, D. E., 7, 28
Jones, D. R., 32, 33, 42, 44
Jones, H. J., 32, 44
Jones, Michael, 158, 180, 226
Joraschky, P., 10, 28
Jung, Carl G., 105, 106, 107, 117

K

Kalmar, P., 4, 29
Katz, J., 4, 26
Keleman, Stanley, 100, 102
Keller, S. E., 182
Kelly, Grace, xviii
Kerekjarto, Margit von, 10, 28, 56, 86, 93, 186, 201, 226
Kiecolt-Glaser, J. K., 159, 180, 181
Kierkegaard, Soren, xxiii
Kiloh, Leslie G., 178, 179
Kimball, C. P., 5, 8, 22, 24, 28
Kindt, W., 198, 201
Klein, Melanie, 213, 223
Klein, M. D. 6, 30
Klekotka, S. J., 234
Klussmann, Rudolph, 68, 69, 82, 83
Knapp, P. H., 227, 228
Koch, U., 186, 200
Koerfer, A., 196, 201
Köhle, Karl, 10, 28, 184, 190, 191, 201, 202, 226
Kornemann, J., 6, 26
Kornfeld, D. S., 8, 27
Krebber, H. J., 4, 29
Kris, E., 213, 223
Kronfol, Z., 177, 181
Kubb, Rosie, 180
Kübler-Ross, E., 92, 93
Küchler, Thomas, 85, 92, 93, 226
Kune, G., 239

L

Labov, W., 188, 201
Lacan, 220
Lambert, F., 32, 45
Lamprecht, K., 8, 28
Langholz, B., 180
Latane, B., 32, 44
Laube, J., 32, 44
Laudenslager, Mark, xx
Lazarus, Leslie, 178, 179
Lempp, F., 14, 26
LeShan, Lawrence, 50, 55
Levine, S., 58, 66
Levy, S. M., 160, 181
Lidz, R. W., 119, 136
Lidz, T., 119, 136
Lifton, R. J., 41, 44
Lindemann, E., 10, 26
Lindstrom, B., 32, 33, 43, 44
Linn, B. S., 177, 181
Linn, M. W., 177, 181
Linnemann, Ebbe, xxi, 226
Lipowsky, Z. J., 10, 25, 28
Lippmann, M., 181
Litwin, A., 180
Loewenstein, R. M., 213, 223
Lubin, J. H., 180
Luckhurst, Elizabeth, 179, 180
Lundin, T., 32, 33, 43, 44
Lunn, D., 175, 181
Lushene, R. E., 164, 169, 171, 183
Luck, P. W., 232
Lützenkirchen, N. J., 8, 22, 28
Lynch, J. J., 161, 181

M

McCammond, S. L., 32, 44
McClelland, David, xx
MacGregor, Governor, 222
McNeil, D. R., 175, 181
Maddox, J., 161, 182
Mahler, Margaret S., 214, 223
Mahoney, Diane, 179

Index (by author)

Malm, J. R., 8, 27
Maluish, A. M., 181
Marek, P., 180
Marsh, J., 6, 29
Mason, J. W., 166, 182
Matt, E., 188, 200
Matthiesen, S. B., 41, 42, 44
Mead, J. H., 215
Mechanic, D., 178, 182
Medawar, J. S., 223
Medawar, P. B., 207, 223
Meffert, H. J., 4, 7, 27, 28, 29, 30
Meng, H., 46, 55
Menninger, Karl A., xiv
Messner, Reinhold, 97, 102
Meyer, A. E., xiv, 10, 28
Meyerowitz, B. E., 59, 66
Meyerson, A. T., 182
Midelfort, C. F., 119, 136
Miles, M. S., 32, 33, 39, 42, 43, 44
Miller, Alice, 95, 103
Miller, B., 232
Minor, M. J., 66
Mirsky, I. A., 119, 136
Mitchell, Jeffrey T., 31, 43, 45, 226
Mölen, K., 8, 24, 25, 27, 29
Mohr, Fritz, xiii
Mohrmann, Klaus, 97
Monro, J. L., 6, 29
Montgomery, Dorothy Adams, xxvi
Morris, T., 160, 180
Mostyn-Aker, P., 32, 44
Mudd, M. C., 186, 202
Müller, H., 27, 29
Murphy, W., 119, 135
Murray, J. R., 66

N

Najman, J. M., 58, 66
Nelder, J. A., 179
Nelson, David, 179
Nelson, M., 165, 182

Nelson, Peggy, 179
Nemetz, S. J., 227
Neumann, C., 196, 201
Nie, N. H., 35, 45
Nilsson-Schonesson, L., 69, 84
Nordmeyer, J., 186, 201
Nordmeyer, J. P., 201
Norton, J., 140, 153, 154, 156
Nothdurft, W., 188, 201

O

O'Donnell, M., 160, 182

P

Patterson, T., 181
Pavlov, Ivan P., xiii, 119, 205, 209, 210, 211
Penn, G. M., 181
Penny, Ronald, 158, 166, 180, 183, 226
Pericles, 95
Perls, F. S., 100, 103
Pettingale, K. W., 160, 182
Petts, V., 180
Petzold, H., 91, 93
Piaget, Jean, 125
Pine, F., 223
Polonius, M. J., 4, 26
Porritt, Don W., 158, 161, 163, 169, 179, 180, 182
Power, P., 108, 117
Pratt, L., 186, 202
Priebe, K., 7, 28
Prüssmann, K., 30

Q

Quasthoff, U. M., 188, 189, 201
Quasthoff-Hartmann, U. M., 201

R

Rabiner, C. J., 7, 29
Rad, M. v., 49, 55
Radloff, L. S., 174, 182
Raphael, B., 32, 33, 39, 42, 45
Raskin, M. J., 182
Raspe, H. H., 185, 186, 187, 201, 202
Ratsak, G., 86, 93
Rawlinson, M., 6, 7, 8, 22, 25, 26
Read, Herbert, 229
Reader, G. G., 186, 202
Reich, G., 74, 83
Reimer, C., 6, 27, 29, 30
Reshauer, xiv
Rice, J., 180
Richardson, H. B., 119, 136
Richter, H. E., 10, 26
Rodewald, G., 3, 4, 29, 30
Rodgers, W. L., 57, 66
Rogentine, G. M., 88, 93
Roose, L. J., 140, 154, 156
Ross, J. K., 6, 7, 29

S

Sakinofsky, I., 10, 29
Sanford, B., 140, 156
Scheld, H., 29
Scherg, H., 160, 182, 234
Schilder, P., 141, 155
Schleifer, S. J., 161, 177, 182, 183
Schlepper, M., 27
Schlien, B., 181
Schmidt, Carl, xiii
Schoeder, H. A., 119, 135
Schur, M., 156
Sebeok, Th., 218, 223
Seidl, O., 73, 74, 83
Selg, H., 10, 27
Selye, Hans, xiii, xiv
Sheehan, M., 232
Sheil, A., 178, 183
Siefen, G., 27
Siegal, S., 166, 183

Siegrist, J., 186, 187, 190, 200, 202
Silva Jr., J., 181
Simons, C., 190, 201
Singer, J., 104, 108, 116, 117
Singh, B., 32, 45
Siris, S. G., 183
Siskin, B., 232
Smith, J., 232, 234
Smith, K., 234
Smith, T. L., 181
Spaeth, L., 10, 29
Spector, Novera Herbert, xx
Spehr, W., 4, 29
Speicher, C. E., 181
Speidel, Hubert, 3, 4, 6, 7, 26, 27, 28, 29, 30, 226
Spielberger, C. D., 164, 169, 171, 183
Spreen, O., 10, 30
Stanley, J. C., 63, 66
Stanton, B. A. 6, 7, 30
Starling, 206
Steele, J. H., 119, 135
Steiger, Th. S., 74, 83
Stein, M., 182, 183
Steinbrenner, K., 35, 44
Steinmann, G., 186, 201
Stephens, P. M., 223
Stierlin, H., 132, 183
Stoeckle, D., 186, 202
Stotland, E., 108, 117
Stout, J. C., 181
Strain, E. C., 181
Surtees, P. G., 167, 180
Szklo, M., 161, 181

T

Tarr, K. L., 181
Taub-Bynum, E., 106, 117
Taylor, A. W., 32, 33, 45
Tee, D. E. H., 182
Templer, D. I., 169, 171, 183
Tennant, Christopher, 158, 165, 179, 183
Thomas, Lewis, xiv

Index (by author)   249

Thornton, J. C., 182
Thyholdt, Reidar, 31, 226
Titus, M. P., 32, 44
Tolstoi, Leo, 99, 103
Toporek, J. D., 180
Troup, S. P., 156

U

Uexküll, Jakob von, 212, 223, 224
Uexküll, Thure von, 203, 210, 223, 226

V

Valent, P., 32, 44
Van Gogh, Vincent, xxi-xxii
Vargiu, J., 105, 117
Vollerts, A., 6, 26

W

Waitzkin, H. J., 186, 202
Wallis, C., 161, 183
Walter, J., 8, 28
Walter, P. J., 5, 30
Waltz, E. M., 5, 10, 30
Wardwell, W., 3, 26, 227, 228, 229, 230, 231 232
Watson, M., 160, 178, 183
Weakland, H., 135
Weber, G., 183
Weimer, E., 69, 84
Weinel, E., 80, 84
Weiner, H., 158, 179
Weingarten, E., 188, 200
Weinger, H., 224
Weinhold, M., 234
Weisaeth, L., 32, 45
Weisman, 65
Weisman, A. D., 140, 141, 148, 150, 156
Weiss, E., 191, 202

Weizsäcker, Viktor von, 47, 48, 52, 53, 54, 55, 118, 205
Wells, John, 179
Wesiack, W., 210, 223
Wessel, M., 4, 27
Westphale, C., 191, 202
Wheeler, L., 32, 44
Wichelhaus, D. P., 83
Wiley, J. A., 66
Wilkinson, C. B., 32, 39, 42, 45
Willner, A. E., 7, 29
Wilson, S. N., 27
Winnicott, D. W., 214, 215, 216, 220, 224
Wirsching, B., 160, 183
Wirsching, M., 160, 183
Withey, S. B., 57, 65
Wolf, xiv
Wolf, S., 119, 135
Wyss, xiv

Y

Yamauchi, Y., 180
Young, M., 161, 183

Z

Zerssen, D. von, 10, 28
Ziegler, J. B., 166, 183
Zimmerman, R. R., 223
Zorn, F., 54, 55
Zurcher, L. A., 32, 45
Zyzanski, S. J., 6, 30

Index (by subject)

A

adaptation, emotional, 8, 21
adjustment, psychological, 8-9, 17-18, 23
aggression, 80, 203, 211, 222; see also drives, aggressive
AIDS, xxv, 68-82
   counselling, 74-79
   diagnosis, 70, 74, 76, 78, 79
   fear of, 68, 75, 81
   in handicapped, 73, 75
      hemophiliacs, 71
      homosexuals, 71, 73, 75
      i.v. drug-dependents (drug-addicts), 71, 72, 73, 75
   sexual behavior, 71, 72, 74, 76, 77, 78
   social reaction to, 73, 75
      isolation, 75
      rejection, 73
   testing, 74, 75, 76-78
      and counselling, 76-78
alcoholism, xxii
"alexithymia", 49-50
alienation, xx
aneurysmectomy, 9
anger, 32, 115, 160
   Cortauld Emotional Control Suppression of Anger subscale, 160
Antarctica, 33
anxiety, xx, 8, 10, 11, 19, 126, 152, 154, 218, 222; see also, fear
   denial of, 8
   in pre- and post-operative patients, 19, 22
   in rescue workers, 32, 35, 36, 37, 38, 40, 41
appendectomy, 192
archetypal context, 106
asthma, 126
Australia, 162, 172
   Australian Veterans' Health Studies, 174
Austria, 96

B

B-cells, 162, 164, 165, 167, 169
bereavement, 161-178
   and physiological and psychological responses, 162-178
   and spouses' mortality rate, 161
   Bereavement Project, 162-178
Bible, 95
biochemistry of emotions, xi
biofeedback, xx
biopsychosocial interactions, xxvi
Bodily Changes in Pain, Hunger, Fear and Rage, xiii
brain tumor, 142-143; see also cancer
breast tumors, xi, 160; see also cancer
burns, 59

C

cancer, xi, xiv-xv, xvi, xviii, xix, xxv, 46-54, 56, 59, 82, 85,105, 111, 159-160
  breast, 56, 59, 63-64, 88, 113, 160-161, 178
    anger suppression and, 160, 161
  carcinoma, 46-47, 49, 54
  leukemia, 142, 169
    monocytic, 144, 147
    myeloblastic, 143
    myeloid, 59
  multiple glioma, 142
  patients, psychotherapy with, 47-54, 85-93
  treatment of,
    chemotherapy, 59, 64, 90
    psychotherapy, 46-54, 85-93
    radiotherapy, 64, 90
    surgery, 64, 90
cardiac
  arrhythmias, 15-16, 23
  paroxysmale tachycardia, 192
  surgery, 3-26
    and employment after, 6-7
    and rehabilitation, psychological and social, 3-26
    aneurysmectomy, 9
    coronary artery bypass surgery (CABS), 6, 9, 59
    heart (coronary) valve correction, 6
      replacement, 7-8, 59
    post-operative difficulties, 4
    psychotherapeutic help after, 5-6, 22
chemical processes,
  intercellular, 205, 206
  intracellular, 205, 206
Cherokee Indians, 111
child development, see psychological development
circulation system, 3
communication, therapeutic 51, 185-199
conditioned reflex, xiii, 210-211
conscious vs. unconscious, 142
coping, 94
  counterphobic mechanism for, 144, 152
  in illness, 79, 107-108, 116, 144
  patterns
    of cardiac patients, 8
    of rescue workers, 43
  styles and strategies, 75, 108, 160
  techniques, xx
cortisol, 162, 166

D

death and dying, xxvi, 12-13, 23, 41, 48, 68, 70, 75, 79, 80, 82, 87, 90, 91, 95-102, 113, 115-116, 137-144, 146-155
  acceptance of, 109
  attitudes towards, 139-140, 142-144, 146-150
  bereavement, 158-159, 161, 162-178
  courage in the face of, 95, 150
  definitions, 137-138
  denial of, 142, 143, 148-151, 155
    "induction of denial", 151-155
  in scholarly literature and fiction, 97-102, 138-148
  interpersonal vs. intrapersonal factors, 140-141, 150
  near-death experiences, 100, 102
  the role of the family, 115-116, 137, 143, 151
  spiritual aspects, 95, 100-102
  Templer Death Anxiety Scale, 169, 171
Death and Neurosis, 101

Death Be Not Proud, 142
The Death of Ivan Illich, 99
defense mechanisms, 8, 22, 69, 73, 74, 90, 91, 145; see also coping
   avoidance, 149
   denial, 73, 90, 92, 142, 148-151, 154, 155
   displacement, 149
   projective identification, 73
   regression, 145
   repression, 87-88, 154
   splitting, 73
dependency, 8
depressive moods/attitudes, 10, 23
depression, xx, 8, 75, 78, 79, 92, 131, 144, 169, 171, 174, 177
   treatment of, xx
diabetes, 119, 126
dialysis, 59, 130, 131
disorder, see also illness
   affective disorder, 134
   psychophysiological disorders, 134
   neurotic disorder, 134
doctor-patient interaction, see patient-physician relationships,
dopamine, 162, 166
dreams, 46, 47, 48, 81, 106, 146-147
drives, 212
   aggressive, 211-213, 215, 217
   "death drive", 213
   libidinous, libidinal, 213, 216, 217; see also drives, sexual
   physiological, 214, 216
   psychological, 204, 206
   psychosomatic, 216
   sexual, 214, 217
   social, 216
   somato-psychological, 206

E

EEG, 96
ego, 69, 70, 73, 79, 104, 139, 147, 148, 152, 155
ego-fragmentation, 51
ego-strength, 142, 149
embryos, mammalian, 212
emotional
   adaptation, 8, 21
   attachments, 155
   attitudes towards death, 139-140, 142-144, 146-150
   changes and disturbances, post-operative, 9, 12-14, 17, 21-25
   complaints, 18, 21
   Cortauld Emotional Control scale, 160
   instability/stability, 11, 13, 18
   problems and recovery after cardiac surgery, 5-6, 21-25
   reactions following a disaster, 31-43
   strain/tension/stress/distress, 12, 22, 24, 31, 159-161
      physiological effects of, xi, 159-161
   well-being, 9
emotions and feelings, xi
   anger, 32, 115, 160
   anxiety, 32, 35, 36, 37, 38, 40, 41, 78, 79, 160, 218, 222; see also fear
   effects of
      on digestive system, xiii
      endocrine system, xi, xiii, 177-178
      immune system, xi, 160-161
      nervous system, xiii
   envy, 80
   fear, 68, 69, 70, 73, 75, 81, 87-88, 90, 91, 144
   frustration, 32, 35, 38, 41, 42; 115, 197

Index (by subject)

grief, 158
guilt, 69, 70, 73, 88-89, 153, 154, 220
hate, 222
helplessness, 32, 35, 36, 38, 42, 68, 73, 75, 81, 92
hopelessness, 36, 38, 42, 75, 81, 108
love, 222
rage, 79, 80
sadness, 32, 37
endocrinological functions and variables, 162-166
epilepsy, xxii
ethical principles in psychotherapy, 85-93
autonomy, 86, 89
benevolence, 86, 92, 93
justice, 87
nihil-nocere, 87, 89, 92
responsibility, 87, 89
truthfulness, 87, 92
European Ein Verdin movement, xii

F

family, 104-116, 118-134
genograms, 105, 109, 110, 112, 114, 126, 133
the role in patient's
coping with illness, 90, 111, 119, 121, 122, 123-131, 133-134
death and dying, 115-116, 137, 139
illness, 119, 132-133
recovery, 7, 16
systematic view of, 122-126, 133-134
affectivity, 122-125
boundaries, 122-124
communication, 122-124, 129
leardership, 122-124
task and goal performance, 122-125

Family Medicine, 119
fear, 68, 69, 72, 73, 75, 81, 87-88, 90, 91, 144; *see also* anxiety
feedback, 206
food poisoning, imaginary, xvii
Freiburger Personality Inventory (FPI), 9-10, 20
Psychosomatic Disturbances scale, 10
From Dream to Discovery, xiii
frustration, 32, 35, 38, 41, 42, 115, 197

G

gastrectomy, 59
genetic codes, 209
genograms, 105, 109, 110, 112, 114, 126, 133
Germany, 6, 7
Gestalt-therapy, 86, 100
Gestalt-Therapy Verbatim, 100-101
Giessen Test (GT), 10
Basic Mood scale, 10
Social Resonance scale, 10
grief, 158
guilt, 69, 70, 73, 88-89, 153, 154, 220

H

Hamilton Depression Scale, 169, 171, 174
handicapped, 73, 75
Harvard University, 142
healing and healers, natural; *see also* illness, treatment
biofeedback, xx
diviner, 88
herbs, 111
laying on of hands, 111
meditation, 109, 113
prayer, 109-111
visualization, 109

heart, *see also* cardiac
 attack (infarction), 3, 96
 paroxysmale tachycardia, 192
 surgery, *see* cardiac surgery
hemophilia, 71
hierarchy of living matter, 120-121
HIV, *see* AIDS
Hodgkin's disease, 56
homosexuals, 71, 73, 75; *see also* sexual behavior
Hopkins Symptoms Checklist (HSCL), 33
hormones, 159, 161, 162, 166, 167, 209
 cortisol, 162, 166
 dopamine, 162, 166
 serotonin, 162, 166
 thyroid, 162
 triiodothyronine, 166
 thyroxine, 166
hypertension, 192
hypertrophic realism, 47, 49, 52
hypnosis, xiv
 and pain relief in cancer patients, 53, 115
 and wart removal, xiv
hypochondria, 8
hysteria, xviii, 8

I

ileostomy, 59, 128
illness, xix, xxvi, 185
 attitudes to, 75
 cardiac, xxv, 3-26
 causes, 158
  psychosocial factors, xi, xvii
 chronic, 22, 26, 118
 coping with, 75, 79, 107-108
 diagnosis of, xv, xvii, xviii, xix, 70, 74, 76, 78, 79
  patients' reactions to, xvii, xix, 70, 149
 families' roles in, 90, 111, 119, 121, 122, 123-134
 incurable, 94-102; *see also* terminal
 individual illnesses
  allergies, 165
  asthma, 126
  cancer, xi, xiv-xv, xvi, xviii, xix, xxv, 46-54, 56, 59, 85, 105
  cardiovascular, 161
  cerebrovascular, 161
  diabetes, 119, 126
  epilepsy, xxii
  hemophilia, 71
  Hodgkin's disease, 56
  hypertension, 192
  multiple sclerosis, 113
  paroxysmale tachycardia, 192
  syphilis, 68
  ulcerative colitis, 126, 127
 mental, xxi-xxiii, 68, 118; *see also* psychosis; schizophrenia and creativity, xxii-xxiv, 49
 prognosis, 192, 196
 psychogenic, xvii-xviii
 psychosomatic aspects of, xxv, 3, 10, 52, 118-119, 126, 160
 social reaction to, 73
 terminal, 105; *see also* incurable
 treatment of, xx, 64, 185, 196; *see also* healing, natural; psychotherapy; surgery
  antibiotics, 131
  dialysis, 59, 130, 131
  painkillers, 153
  sedatives, 153
 veneral, 68
immune system, immunity, xi, xiv, xx, xxv, 158-178, 218; *see also* psychoimmunology; psychoneuroimmunology
 antibodies, 159, 166

Index (by subject)

bereavment and, 161, 162-178
  endocrine and, 177-178
  loneliness and, 161
  marital disharmony and, 159
  stress and, 159-161
  immunosuppression, 162, 165, 166, 177-178
  B-cell function, 162, 164, 165, 167, 169
  T-cell function, 162, 163, 164, 165, 167, 169, 175, 177
Index Medicus, 58
infarctus, *see* heart attack
International Consortium for the Study of Neurological and Psychological Reactions to Cardiac Surgery, 4
intestinal bypass surgery, 59

J

Jackson Research Form, 165
  Affiliation, Autonomy, and Social Desirability Scales, 164-165

L

leukemia, 142, 169
  monocytic, 144, 147
  myeloblastic, 143
  myeloid, 59
libido, libidinal, libidinous, 152, 154, 155, 213, 216, 217, 222
light, experience of, 100, 102, 111, 113
Living Your Dying, 100
lymphocytes, 159, 165

M

malignant nodules/tumors, *see* cancer

marital disharmony and immune dysfunctions, 159
mastectomy, 64
medical
  care, 56, 59
  costs of, xvi
  insurance, xvi
  rehabilitation, 14-16
  sociology, 185-186
  therapy, impact on quality of life (QOL), 56-65
    definitions, 56-57
    impact of health on, 58
    measurements of, 57, 65
    social indicators of, objective and subjective, 57-61
    studies on, 57-65
  treatment, xx, 64, 185, 196; *see also* healing, natural; psychotherapy; surgery
Medicare, xvi
MEDLARS, 58
meditation, 109, 113
The Medusa and the Snail, xiv
melancholy, xi
methodology, 9-10, 34-35, 163-166, 168-169, 172-175
microvascular bypass surgery, 59
mind, its role in illness and healing, xiii, xvii, xxv; *see also* psychosomatic; psychoimmunology; psychoneuroimmunology
mind/body, *see also* psychosomatic
  connections, xx, xxv
  studies, xii, xiii
Minnesota Multiphasic Personality Inventory (MMPI), 8
morbidity, 158, 163, 172, 174, 175, 176-178
mortality, 3, 94, 161, 162, 163, 172, 175, 176-178
  and bereavement, 162-178
multiple sclerosis, 113

N

narcissism, primary, 212, 213
National Collaborative Leukemia Study, 169
NATO, 31
neuroendocrinology, 177; see also, psychoimmunology; psychoneuroimmunology
neuropeptides, 159
neurosis, 49, 52
neurotic
    fears, 22
    tendencies, 18
Norway, Norwegian, 31, 34

O

oedipal conflict, 145
oncology, see cancer

P

pain, 52-53, 61, 101, 106, 115, 154, 218
paranormal, 106, 111
paroxysmale tachycardia, 192
patient-physician relationships, xiv-xvi, 72, 78, 184-199
    self-responsibility of a patient, 195
Patients Have Families, 119
persona (according to Jung), 105-106
prayer, 107, 109-111, 144
Psi-System, 204, 206
psyche vs. soma, 203
psychic, see paranormal psychoanalysis, 47, 49, 54, 138, 139, 143-147, 153-154, 196, 197
psychoimmunology, 178; see also psychoneuroimmunology
psychological
    adjustment, 8-9, 17-18, 23
    development, 213-216, 219-220
    difficulties
        after cardiac surgery, 5, 21-25
        of breast cancer patients, 64
        of rescue workers, 32-34
    disturbances and problems, 3, 22, 25
    drives, 204, 206
    processes, 206, 208
        and biological processes, 206
    scales
        AMDP/HRPD, 10, 13
        Cohen's polarity profile, 10
        Cortauld Emotional Control scale, 160
            Suppression of Anger sub-scale, 160
        Giessen Test (GT), 10
            Basic Mood scale, 10
            Social Resonance scale, 10
        Freiburger Personality Inventory (FPI), 9-10, 20
            Psychosomatic Disturbances scale, 10
        Hamilton Depression Scale, 169, 171, 174
        Hopkins Symptoms Checklist (HSCL), 33
        Jackson Research Form, 165
            Affiliation, Autonomy, and Social Desirability Scales, 164-165
        Minnesota Multiphasic Personality Inventory (MMPI), 8
        Saarbruecken Anxiety List (SAL), 10
        self-report depression symptom scale CES-D, 174
        State Trait Anxiety Scale (STAI), 164, 169, 170, 171, 174

Index (by subject)

Templer Death Anxiety
 Scale, 169, 171
Tennant and Andrews Life
 Event Inventory, 165
Psychological Abstracts, 58
The Psychology of Death, 101
psychoneuroimmunology, xii,
 70; *see also* immune system;
 psychoimmunology
psychopathological disturbances and problems
 assessment of, 10, 14
 phobic-hypohondriac attitudes, 14
 post-operative, 4, 7, 9-10,
  13-14, 18, 23
 preoperative, 18
 psycho-organic
  syndrome, 7
 disturbances 14
psychosis, 46, 48, 51, 106, 128,
 131
psychosomatic
 approach, 184-199, 203-204,
  219
 aspects of
  aggressiveness, 218
  illness, 3, 10, 52, 118-119, 126, 160
  complaints, symptoms, and
   disturbances, 10, 11, 20-23, 70
  theory, 204-211
psychotherapy, xxv, 85, 79, 94-102, 196-199
 crisis intervention, 56, 78, 86
 Gestalt-therapy, 86, 100
 family consultation
  therapy, 86
 life-panorama technique,
  86
 psychoanalysis, 47, 49, 54,
  79, 138, 139, 143-147,
  153-154, 196, 197
 libido, libidinal, libidinous,
  152, 154, 155, 213, 216,
  217, 222

oedipal conflict, 145
rational therapy, 54
Rogerian client-centered
 therapy, 196, 197
the role of the unconscious,
 47-48
setting-supportive therapy,
 86
transference, 47, 79-81, 145,
 153, 154
counter-transference, 74,
 79-81, 153, 154
verbal-psychotherapy, 196
with cancer patients, 47-54,
 85-93, 147, 220
 ethical principles and
  issues in, 85-93
  autonomy, 86, 89
  benevolence, 86, 92,
   93
  justice, 87
  nihil-nocere, 87, 89,
   92
  responsibility, 87, 89
  truthfulness, 87, 92
 social resistance to, 54
with AIDS patients, 71, 74-82
with incurably ill patients,
 94-102
with post-operative cardiac
 patients, 5-6, 22
with schizophrenic patients,
 46-52

R

rational therapy, 54
Red Cross, 31, 32, 34-37
rehabilitation, 192
 after cardiac surgery, 3-26
 medical, 14-16
 professional, 16
 psychological and social,
  3-9, 10-14, 17-26
religion, 164, 170

religious
 beliefs, 108
 experiences, 108
 faith, 149
 values, 90, 95-100
rescue workers, 31
 emotional reactions following a disaster, 31-42
  anger, 32
  anxiety and fear, 32, 35, 36, 37, 38, 40, 41
  disbelief, 32
  frustration, 32, 35, 36, 38, 42
  helplessness, 32, 35, 36, 38, 42
  hopelessness, 36, 38, 41
  sadness, 32, 37
 role of group support, 43
 sex differences in rescuers' reactions, 42
 sleep disturbances of, 32, 33, 36, 37
 stress experienced by, 32, 33, 36, 39
Rogerian client-centered therapy, 196, 197

S

Saarbruecken Anxiety List (SAL), 10
The Saturday Review, xii
schizophrenia, 46-47, 49-52, 54, 119, 134
 and oncological diseases, 51
Self, 107
self-report depression symptom scale CES-D, 174
self-responsibility of a patient, 195
semiotics, semiotic processes, 207, 210, 211, 212
The Separation of Lovers, 100
serotonin, 162, 166
sexuality, 68, 69, 75, 80; see *also* sexual behavior
sexual
 behavior, 71, 72, 74
 dysfunctions and problems, 7, 145
Siddartha, 101, 102
social resonance, 11, 21-22
socio-demographic variables, 163-164, 168, 170
socio-psychobiology, 218
soma vs. psyche, 203
somato-psychological
 drive, 206
 process, 205
spinal-cord injury, xxv, 109-111
spiritual dimensions, 104-116; see *also* death and dying, spiritual aspects
 and wholeness, 105
 experience of light, 100, 102, 111, 113
St. Vincent's Hospital, 166
State Trait Anxiety Scale (STAI), 164, 169, 170, 171, 174
statistics, 37-38
 analysis of variance, 19
 BMDP, 175
 cluster analysis, 10, 21, 22
  interactive k-Means cluster analysis, 10
 Fisher exact test, 166
 Mann-Whitney Test, 166
 Multivariate Analysis of Variance (MANOVA), 169
 SPSS, 35
 SPIDA, 175
 unpaired t-tests, 166
 Wilcoxon Sum Rank Test (WSRT), 166
Stay of Execution, 142
stress, 158, see *also* emotional strain/stress
 bereavement and, 161, 162-163
 hormonal response, 168
 immune dysfunction, 159-161

Index (by subject)

natuaral killer cell (NK)
  activity, 159, 160
suicide, 73, 96, 131
Supreme Court, xx
surgery, 59
  appendectomy, 192
  cardiac, 3-26
    aneurysmectomy, 9
    coronary artery bypass
      surgery (CABS), 6, 9, 59
    heart (coronary) valve
      correction, 6
      replacement, 7-8, 59
  gastrectomy, 59
  hip replacement, 59
  intestinal bypass surgery, 59
  ileostomy, 59, 128
  in treatment of cancer, 87-88
    hemi-pelvectomy, 87
    mastectomy, 64, 160
  microvascular bypass
    surgery, 59
  transplant, 178
    and immunosuppression,
      178
    kidney transplant, 59
    liver transplant, 59
Sweden, 34
syphilis, 68
systems theory, 207, 211

T

T-cells, 162, 163, 164, 165,
  166, 167, 169, 175, 178
Templer Death Anxiety Scale,
  169, 171
Tennant and Andrews Life
  Event Inventory, 165
thyroid hormones, 162
  triiodothyronine, 166
  thyroxine, 166
transmission of
  information, 209
  meaning, 210
transpersonal psychology, 104

U

UCLA, xii, xiv, xvi
  School of Medicine, xii
  Task Force on
    Psychoneuroimmunology,
    xii, xix
ulcerative colitis, 126, 127
unconscious, 47-48, 73, 80,
  148, 150
  collective, 105, 106
  vs. conscious, 142
United World Federalists, xii
University of California
  Los Angeles, see UCLA
  San Francisco, Medical
    School at Fresno, xii
USA, 4, 6

V

values, religious, 90, 95-100
  salvation, 95
verbal-psychotherapy, 196
Vietnam, 96
visualization, 109, 115

W

warts, xiv
The Way of an Investigator, xiii
Wisdom of the Body, xiii
World Association of World
  Federalists, xii
Wold Health Organization, 174,
  183

Y

Yale University, Center for
  Epidemiologic Studies, 174

Spiritual Dimensions of Healing
From Native Shamanism to Contemporary Health Care
Stanley Krippner, Ph.D. and Patrick Welch

"Krippner and Welch have written a rare book on the topic of healing—one that is at once warmly objective, scholarly, and based on many personal experiences. The reader is given a fine comparative lattice-work for shamanism and several other systems of healing."
—**Jean Achterberg, Ph.D.**
Author of Imagery in Healing and Woman as Healer

"This book is a treasure trove of insights. Krippner and Welch take their readers on a search for the psychodynamics of healing, for cross-cultural patterns of interactive therapies, and, yes, for the secrets of life itself."
—**Stuart Fischer, M.D.**
The Atkins Center for Complimentary Medicine, New York City

"This book presents a broad and judicial coverage of contemporary spiritual healing. It will be informative for both scholar and layperson."
—**Douglas Price-Williams, Ph.D.**
Emeritus Professor, Departments of Psychiatry and Anthropology, University of California, Los Angeles

$39.95 Cloth (includes audio cassette)
$19.95 Book Only

Alive & Well
A Path for Living in a Time of HIV
Peter A. Hendrickson, Ph.D.

"Here at last is a practical, accessible handbook to help you discover how to apply body-mind-spirit medicine in your own life. I recommend it to all of those with HIV and all others too."
—**Sandra McLanahan, M.D.**
Medical Director, Integral Health Services, Buckingham, Virginia

"A deeply useful book about facing AIDS, written from the heart by an experienced psychologist who has a profound understanding of the integration of yoga and the best of contemporary psychology."
—**Michael Lerner, Ph.D.**
Founder Commonweal Cancer Help Program, Bolinas, California

"A book for our time! Helpful to persons with HIV as well as counselors and care givers in understanding the dynamics of incorporating body, mind, and spirit in the healing process."
—**Dr. Robert L. Polk**
Founder of the Minority AIDS Task Force and Former Director of the Council of Churches of the City of New York

$12.95 Paper • $24.95 Cloth

FRONTIERS OF CONSCIOUSNESS

A SERIES OF BOOKS, MANY ACCOMPANIED BY AUDIO AND/OR VIDEO CASSETTES
Series Editor: Stanley Krippner, Ph.D., California Institute of Integral Studies and Saybrook Institute

NOW AVAILABLE FROM IRVINGTON PUBLISHERS

CONFRONTING LIFE-THREATENING ILLNESS
Mind-Body Approaches
Suzanne R. Engelman, Ph.D., Editor
$19.95 Paper

"This remarkable book explores new perspectives on the emotions, spirituality, and quality of life of those faced with life-threatening illness."
—Stanley Krippner, Ph.D., author of *Spiritual Dimensions of Healing*

OTHER BOOKS AVAILABLE FROM IRVINGTON PUBLISHERS

Shamans of the 20th Century
Ruth-Inge Hienze, Ph.D.
$14.95 Paper • $29.95 Cloth

Spiritual Dimensions of Healing
*Stanley Krippner, Ph.D.
and Patrick Welch*
$39.95 Cloth (includes audio cassette)
$19.95 Book Only

Creative Brainstorms
The Relationship Between
Madness and Genius
Russell R. Monroe, M.D.
$24.95 Cloth

Male Sexual Armor
Erotic Fantasies and Sexual Realities of the Cop on the Beat and the Man in the Street
Patrick Suraci, Ph.D.
$19.95 Cloth

Theory of the Moral Life
John Dewey
$12.95 Paper

Lesbian & Gay Lifestyles
A Guide for Counseling and Education
Natalie Woodman
$14.95 Paper

Alive & Well
A Path for Living in a Time of HIV
Peter A. Hendrickson, Ph.D.
$12.95 Paper • $24.95 Cloth
Audio Cassettes also available:
Guided Imagery Exercises for Healing
$11.00
Hatha Yoga for Health and Relaxation
$14.00

IF NOT AVAILABLE FROM YOUR LOCAL BOOKSELLER ORDER DIRECT FROM:

IRVINGTON PUBLISHERS, INC
195 McGregor St. • Manchester, NH 03102
Phone (603) 669-5933 • Fax (603) 669-7945

ORDER FORM
Irvington Publishers, Inc.
195 McGregor St., Manchester, NH 03102
(603) 669-5933 Fax (603) 669-7945

Shipping Address: Name_____

Address_____

City_____State_____Zip_____

VISA or Mastercard #_____

Exp. Date_____Signature_____

QTY	TITLE	PRICE	TOTAL
		DISCOUNTED SUBTOTAL	
		Tax, Shipping and Handling	
		TOTAL	

U.S., Canada, Mexico shipping & handling, add $4.00 per order. Overseas (via airmail) $10.00 each order. Individuals must include check, money order or credit card information. Libraries and institutions may enclose purchase orders for books and will be billed at current prices less sales discount. Delivery Approx. 4 weeks.

Tax: NY Residents Only (NYC 8.25%)